My Mediterranean Diet Cookbook

Easy Breakfast And Brunch Recipes To Start Each Day

Ben Cooper

Table of contents

6

Mini Frittatas

Preparation time: 5 minutes
Cooking time: 15 minutes
Servings: 12

Ingredients:

1 yellow onion, chopped 1 cup parmesan, graten

1 yellow bell pepper

1 red bell pepper

1 zucchini, chopped

Salt and black pepper to the taste

8 eggs, whisked

A drizzle of olive oil

2 tablespoons chives, chopped

Directions:

1.Heat a pan with the oil over medium-high heat, add the onion, the zucchini and all the ingredients (except the eggs), chives and sauté for 5 minutes stirring often.

2. Divide this mix on the bottom of a muffin pan, pour the eggs mixture on top, sprinkle salt, pepper and the chives and bake at 350 degrees F for 10 minutes.

3.Serve the mini frittatas for breakfast right away.

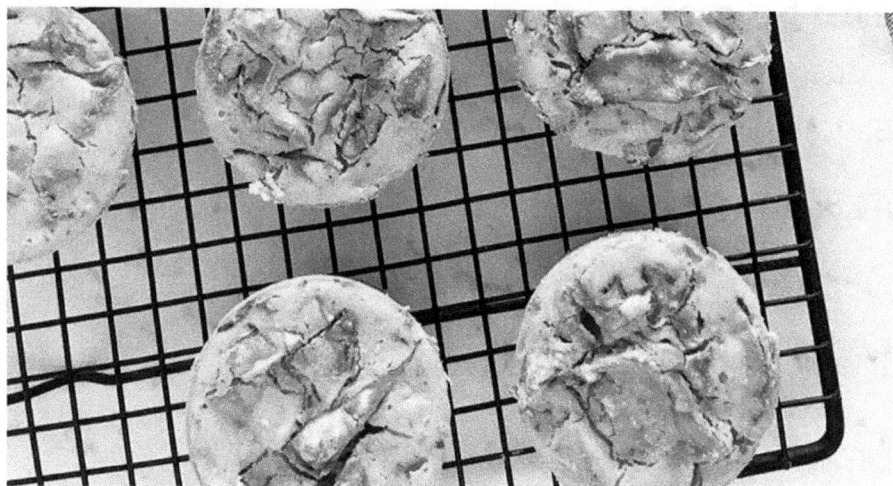

Berry Oats

Preparation time: 5 minutes
Cooking time: 0 minutes
Servings: 2

Ingredients:

½ cup rolled oats 1 cup almond milk
¼ cup chia seeds
A pinch of cinnamon powder
2 teaspoons honey
1 cup berries, pureed
1 tablespoon yogurt

Directions:

1.In a bowl, combine the oats with the milk and the rest of the ingredients except the yogurt, toss, divide into bowls, top with the yogurt and serve cold for breakfast.

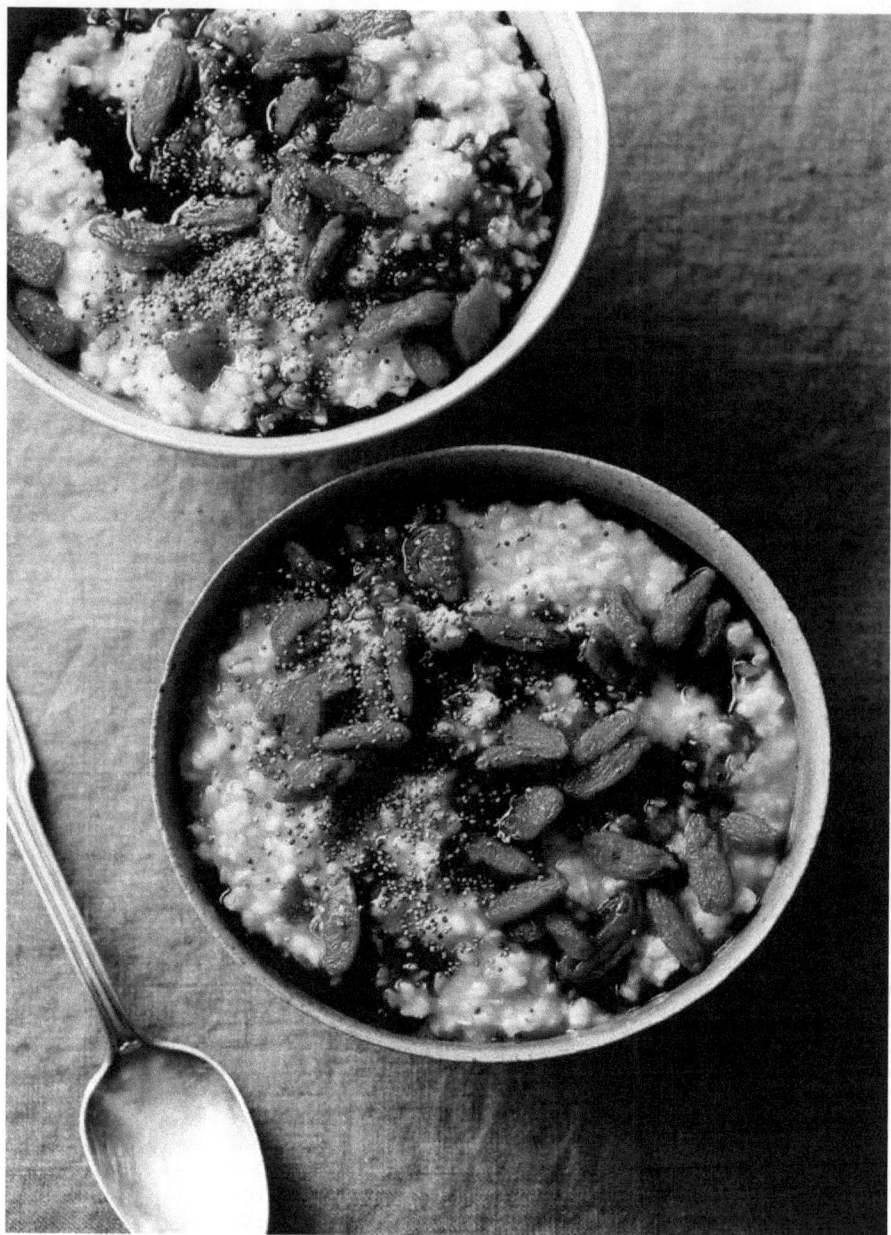

Quinoa and Eggs Pan

Preparation time: 10 minutes
Cooking time: 23 minutes
Servings: 4

Ingredients:

4 bacon slices, cooked and crumbled A drizzle of olive oil
1 small red onion
1 red bell pepper
1 sweet potato, grated
1 green bell pepper
2 garlic cloves, minced
1 cup white mushrooms, sliced
½ cup quinoa
1 cup chicken stock
4 eggs, fried
Salt and black pepper to the taste

Directions:

1.Heat a pan with the oil over medium-low heat, add the onion, garlic, bell peppers, sweet potato and the mushrooms, toss and sauté for 5 minutes.

2.Add the quinoa, toss and cook for 1 more minute.

3.Add the stock, salt and pepper, stir and cook for 15 minutes.

4.Divide the mix between plates, top each serving with a fried egg, sprinkle some salt, pepper, crumbled bacon, and serve breakfast.

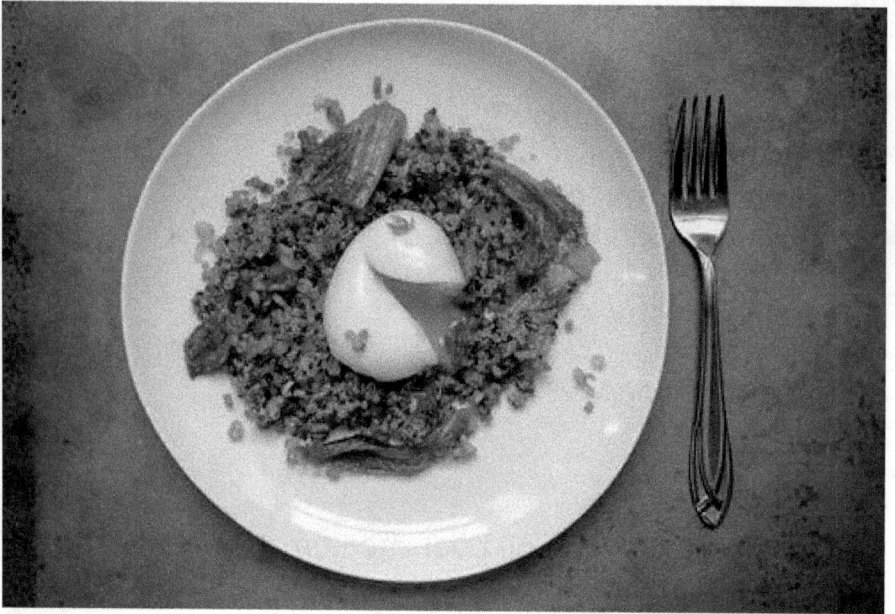

Stuffed Tomatoes

Preparation time: 10 minutes
Cooking time: 15 minutes
Servings: 4

Ingredients:

2 tablespoons olive oil
8 tomatoes, insides scooped
¼ cup almond milk 8 eggs
¼ cup parmesan, grated
Salt and black pepper to the taste
4 tablespoons rosemary, chopped

Directions:

1.Grease a pan with the oil and arrange the tomatoes inside.

2.Crack an egg in each tomato, divide the milk and the rest of the ingredients, introduce the pan in the oven and bake at 375 degrees F for 15 minutes.

3.Serve for breakfast right away.

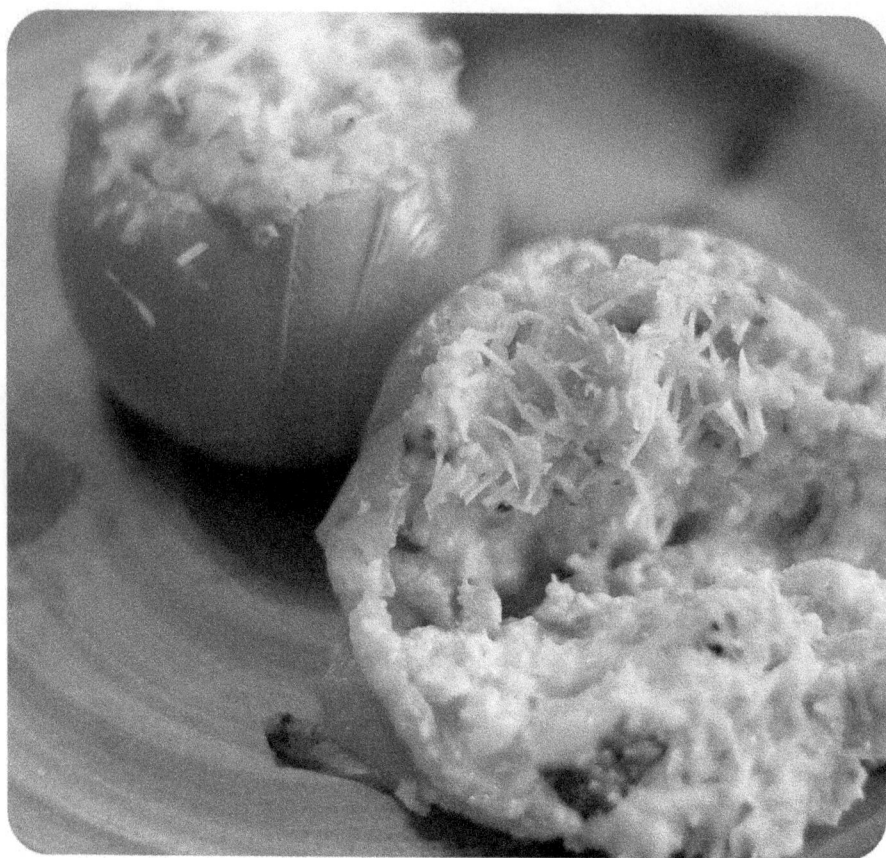

Watermelon "Pizza"

Preparation time: 10 minutes
Cooking time: 0 minutes
Servings: 4

Ingredients:

1 watermelon slice cut 1-inch thick and then from the center cut into 4 wedges resembling pizza slices
6 kalamata olives, pitted and sliced
1-ounce feta cheese, crumbled
½ tablespoon balsamic vinegar 1 teaspoon mint, chopped

Directions:

1.Arrange the watermelon "pizza" on a plate, sprinkle the olives and the rest of the ingredients on each slice and serve right away for breakfast.

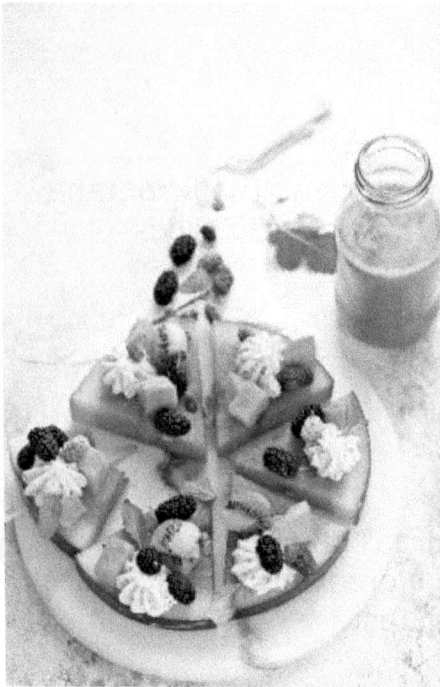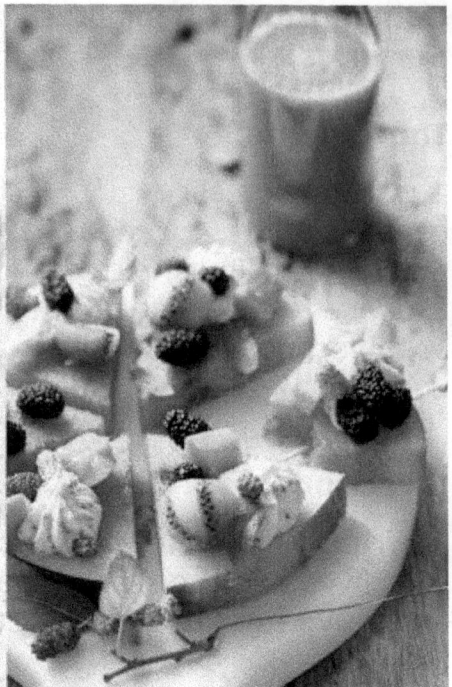

Avocado and Feta Cheese Baked Eggs

Preparation Time: 25 minutes
Cooking Time: 15 minutes
Servings: 2

Ingredients:

Salt and pepper One-quarter of a teaspoon each Eggs, (four)
Feta cheese, three tablespoons
Crumbled finely Avocado, one large, cut into slices
Olive oil, two tablespoons

Directions:

1.Heat the oven to 350. Lay the slices of avocado into two oven-safe personal- sized baking dishes.

2.Crack two of the eggs into each bowl easily, so you do not break the yoke. Add the cheese crumbles and lightly sprinkle pepper and salt in each cup. Bake them for fifteen minutes.

3. Serve

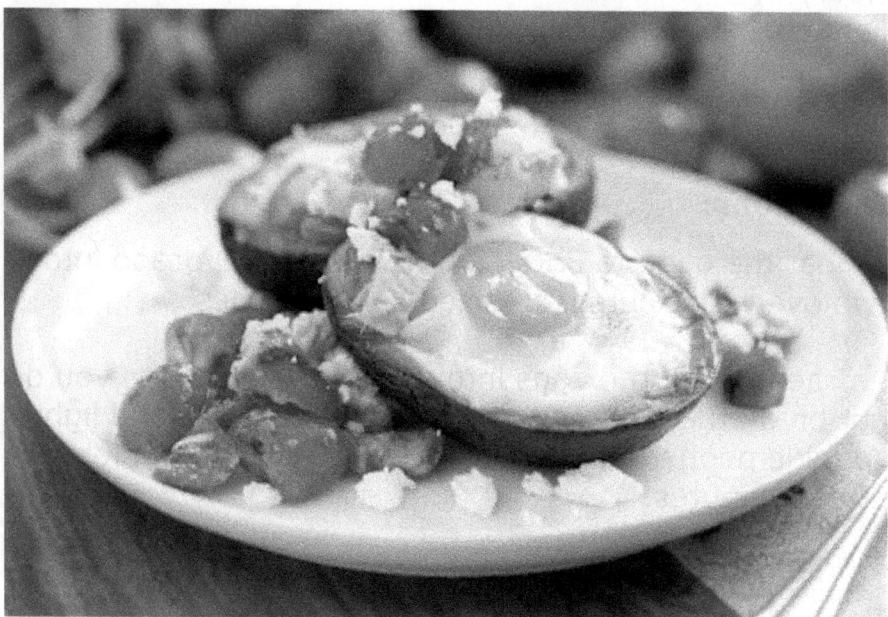

Greek Yogurt Pancakes

Preparation Time: 15 minutes
Cooking Time: 15 minutes
Servings: 6

Ingredients:

Flour, one and one-quarter cup
Blueberries, one-half of a cup, fresh or frozen
Salt, one-quarter of a teaspoon
Baking powder, two teaspoons
Milk, one-half of a cup
Baking soda one teaspoon
Butter three tablespoons
Plain Greek yogurt, one and one-half of a cup
Eggs, three

Directions:

1.Mix the dry ingredients and the wet ingredients separately; leave the blueberries for now.

2.Mix wet and dry ingredients and then gently fold in the blueberries.

3.Top the pancakes with more yogurt and blueberries if desired.

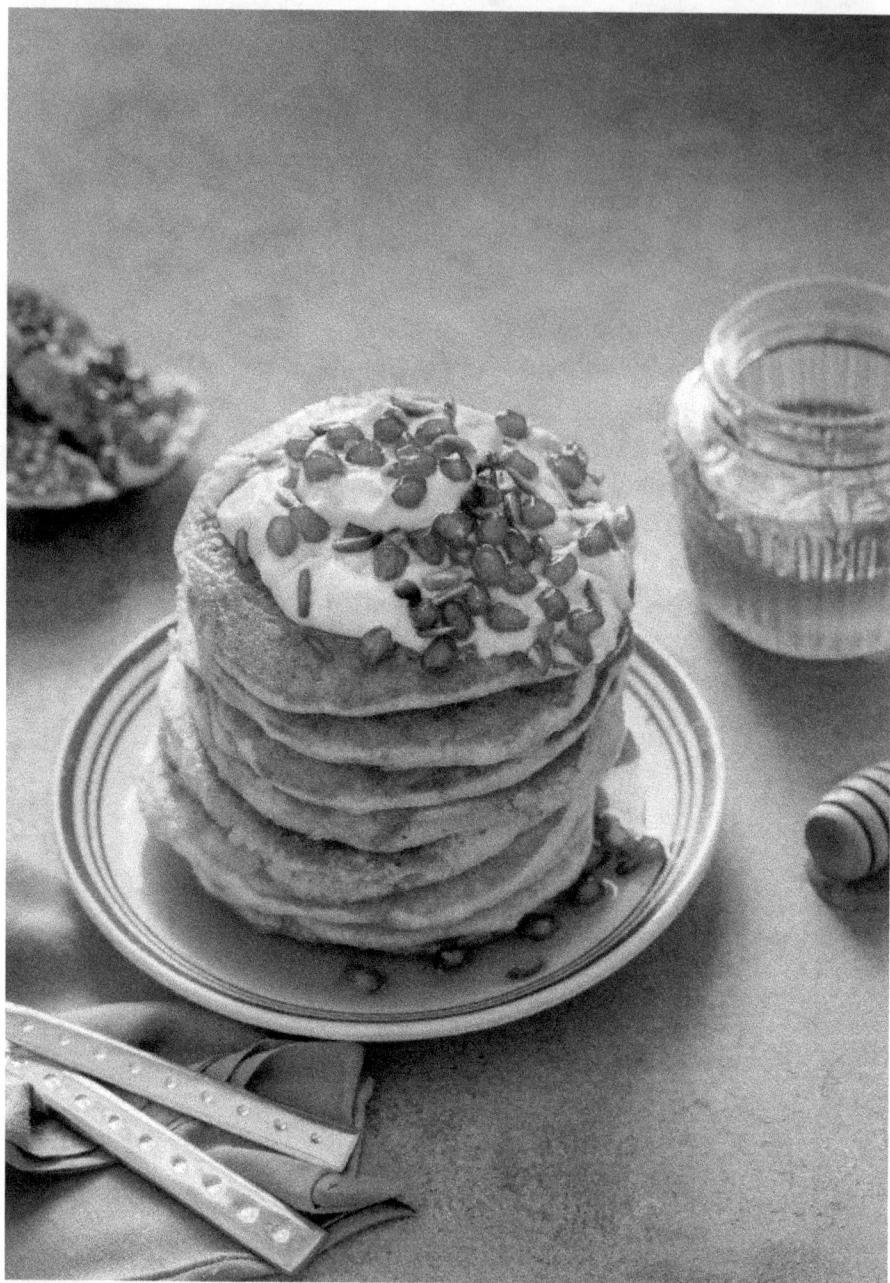

Mediterranean Eggs

Preparation Time: 5 minutes
Cooking Time: 1 hour and 18 minutes
Servings: 6

Ingredients:

Yellow onion, one large, cut in thin slices
Parsley, one-quarter of a cup, chopped finely
Butter, one tablespoon
Sea salt one-quarter of a teaspoon
Olive oil, one tablespoon
Black pepper, one-half of a teaspoon
Garlic, one clove, chopped fine
Feta cheese, three ounces, crumbled small
Tomatoes, one-half of a cup cut in thin slices
Eggs, eight

Directions:

1.Cook the onions in the butter for about ten minutes. Stir in the olive oil, along with the tomatoes and garlic and cook for five more minutes.

2.Lower the heat and break the eggs over the mix, drizzling with pepper, salt, and feta.

3.Cover and cook for ten minutes without stirring over low heat. Sprinkle on the parsley and serve.

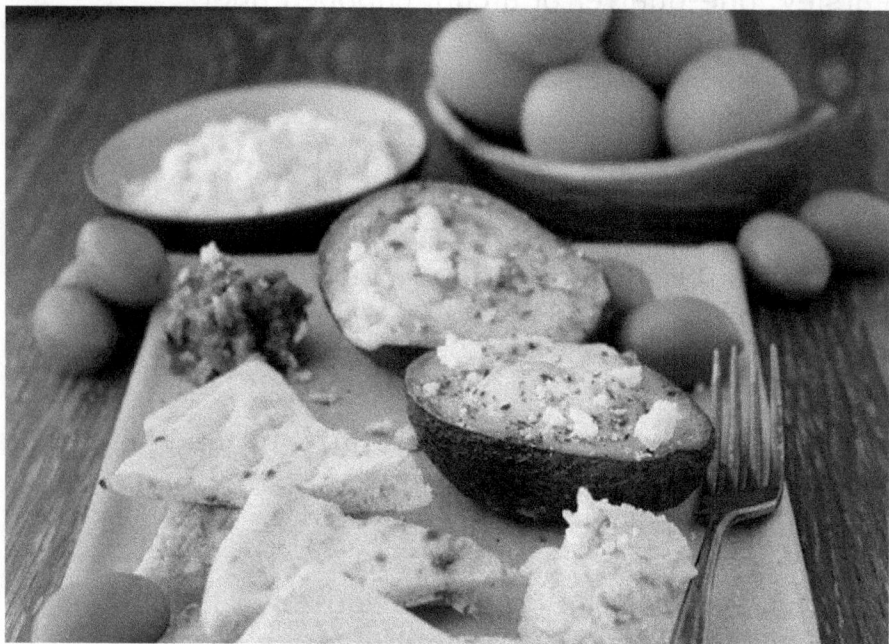

Mediterranean Breakfast Salad

Preparation Time: 30 minutes
Cooking Time: 0 minutes
Servings: 4

Ingredients:

Eggs, four, hard-boiled and sliced in thin slices Lemon
juice, three tablespoons
Arugula, ten cups, washed and dried
Olive oil, two tablespoons
Tomato, one large, cut into eight wedges
Dill, one-half of a cup, chopped finely
Cucumber, one-half of a cup, chopped finely
Almonds, one cup, chopped finely
Quinoa, one cup, cooked and already cooled
Avocado, one large, sliced in thin slices

Directions:

1.Mix the quinoa with the tomatoes, cucumber, and
arugula. Add the salt, pepper, and olive oil; toss lightly.

2.Place the salad mix on four salad plates, arrange the
sliced egg and the avocado slices on top of the salad
mix, and top with the almonds and herbs.

3.Drizzle the lemon juice all over it.

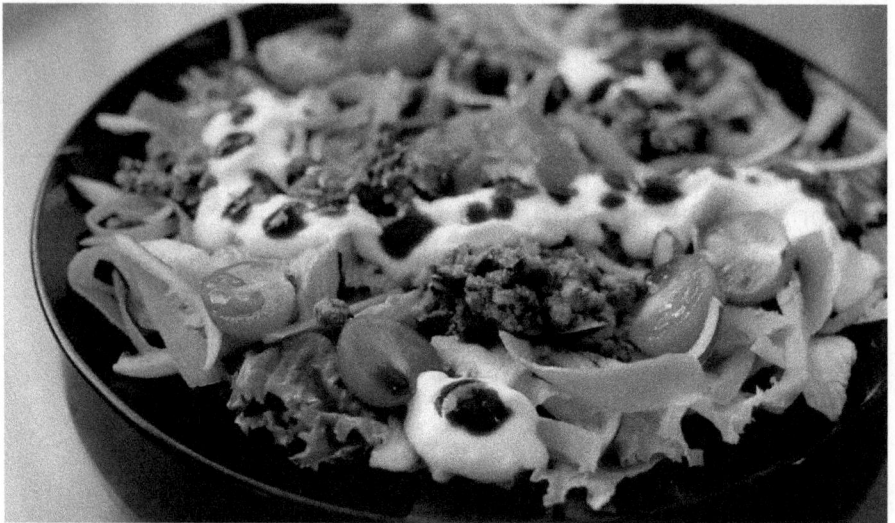

Mushroom and Spinach Omelet

Preparation Time: 3 minutes
Cooking Time: 15 minutes
Servings: 1-2

Ingredients:

Olive oil, one tablespoon
Green onion, one, diced finely
Red onion, one-quarter of a cup, diced finely
Egg, three
Spinach, one and one-half fresh, chopped small
Feta cheese, one-half of a cup, crumbled small
Button mushrooms, five, sliced thinly

Directions:

1.Sauté the onions, mushrooms, and spinach for three minutes in the olive oil and then set them to the side.

2.Pour the well-beaten eggs into the skillet. Cook the eggs for about 3 or 4 minutes until the edges begin to brown.

3.Sprinkle all of the other ingredients onto half of the omelet and fold the other half over the ingredients.

4.Cook the omelet for one minute on each side.

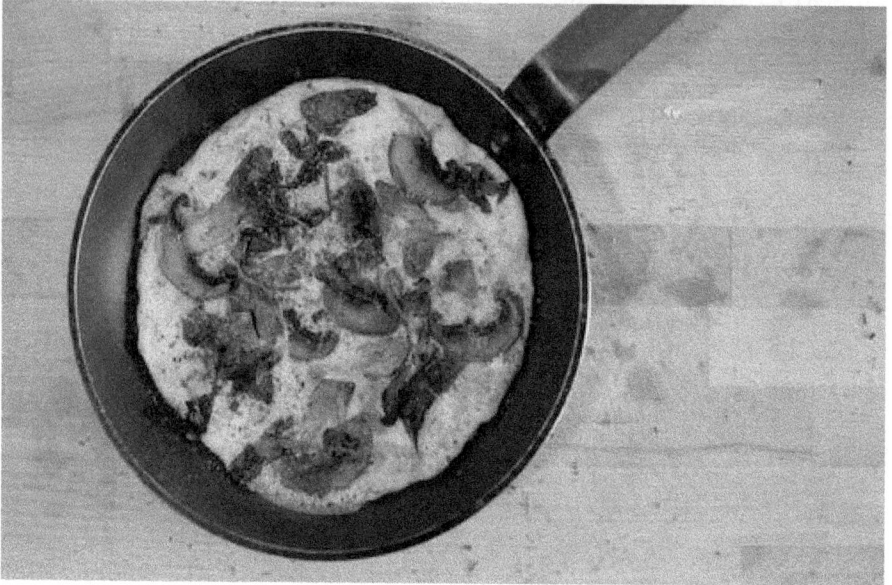

Southwest Tofu Scramble

Preparation Time: 10 minutes
Cooking Time: 20 minutes
Servings: 2

Ingredients:

Kale, two cups, washed, dried, and chopped into small pieces
Eggs, four, beaten well
Red pepper, one-half of one, sliced thinly
Olive oil, two tablespoons
Red onion, one-fourth of one, sliced thinly
Garlic powder, one teaspoon
Turmeric, a quarter teaspoon
Water, just enough to thin ingredients
Chili powder, a quarter teaspoon
Sea salt, one-half teaspoon
Cumin powder, one-half teaspoon

Directions:

1.Make the sauce, mix all of the spices in a bowl, and add just enough water to stir into a sauce-type of consistency.

2.Cook the red pepper, kale, and onion for three to four minutes in the olive oil. Then pour the beaten egg all over the mix in the pan, and cook it until the eggs reach your desired set.

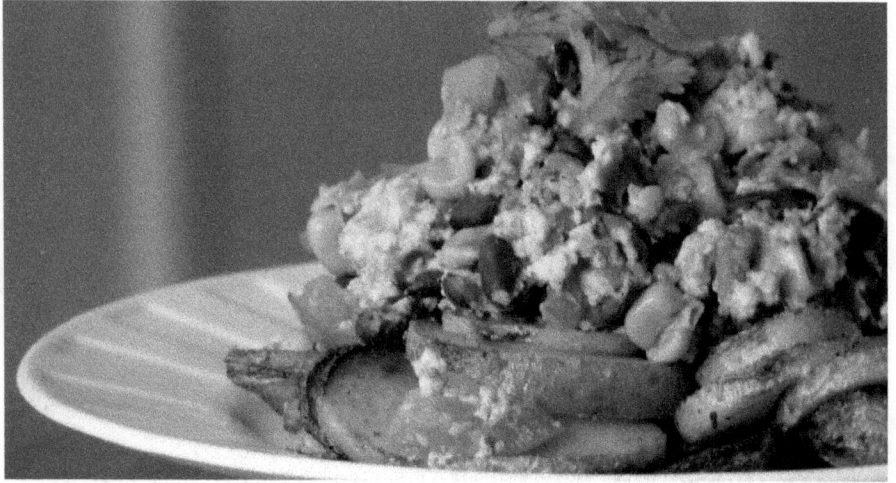

Ricotta & Pear Bake

Preparation Time: 10 minutes
Cooking Time: 15 minutes
Servings: 4

Ingredients:

16 Ounce Whole Milk Ricotta Cheese
2 Eggs, Large
1 Tablespoon Sugar
¼ Cup Whole Wheat Flour
1 Teaspoon Vanilla Extract, Pure
¼ Teaspoon Nutmeg 2 Tablespoon Water
1 Pear, Cored & Diced
1 Tablespoon Honey, Raw

Directions:

1.Heat your oven to 400, and then get out four ramekins that are six ounces each. Grease them with cooking spray.

2.Get out a bowl and beat your eggs, flour, sugar, ricotta, vanilla, and nutmeg together. Spoon this mixture into your ramekins, baking for about twenty-five minutes. The ricotta should be almost set.

3.Remove from the oven, and let it cool.

4.While you make your ricotta get out a saucepan and place it over medium heat. Simmer your pears in water for ten minutes. They should soften, and then remove them from heat.

5.Stir your honey in, and then serve the ricotta ramekins topped with your cooked pears.

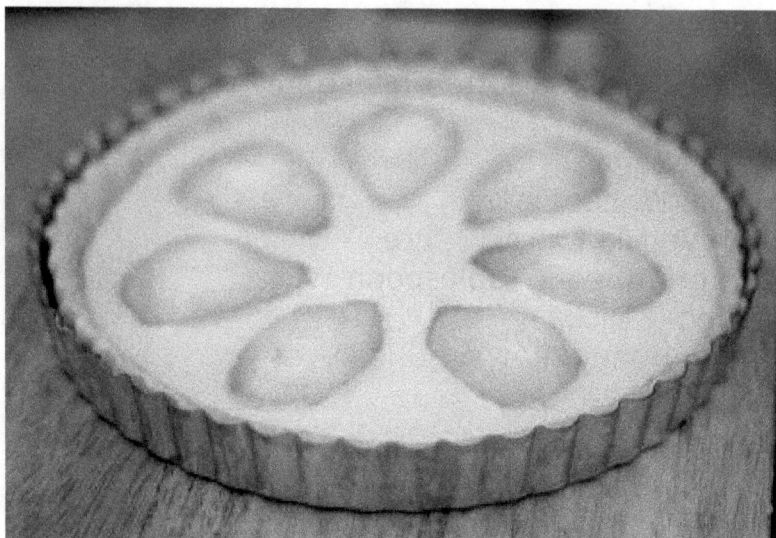

Fruit Bulgur

Preparation Time: 5 minutes
Cooking Time: 10 minutes
Servings: 5

Ingredients:

2 Cups Milk, 2%
1 ½ Cups Bulgur, Uncooked
½ Teaspoon Cinnamon
2 Cups Dark Sweet cherries, Frozen 8 Figs, Dried &
Chopped
½ Cup Almonds, Chopped
¼ Cup Mint, Fresh & Chopped
½ Cup Almonds, Chopped Warm 2% Milk to Serve

Directions:

1.Get out a medium saucepan and combine your water, cinnamon, bulgur and milk. Stir it once and bring it just to a boil. Once it begins to boil then cover it, and then reduce your heat to medium-low.
2.Allow it to simmer for ten minutes. The liquid should be absorbed.

3.Turn the heat off, but keep your pan on the stove. Stir in your frozen cherries. You don't need to thaw them, and then ad din your almonds and figs. Stir well before covering for a minute.

4.Stir your mint in, and then serve with warm milk drizzled over it.

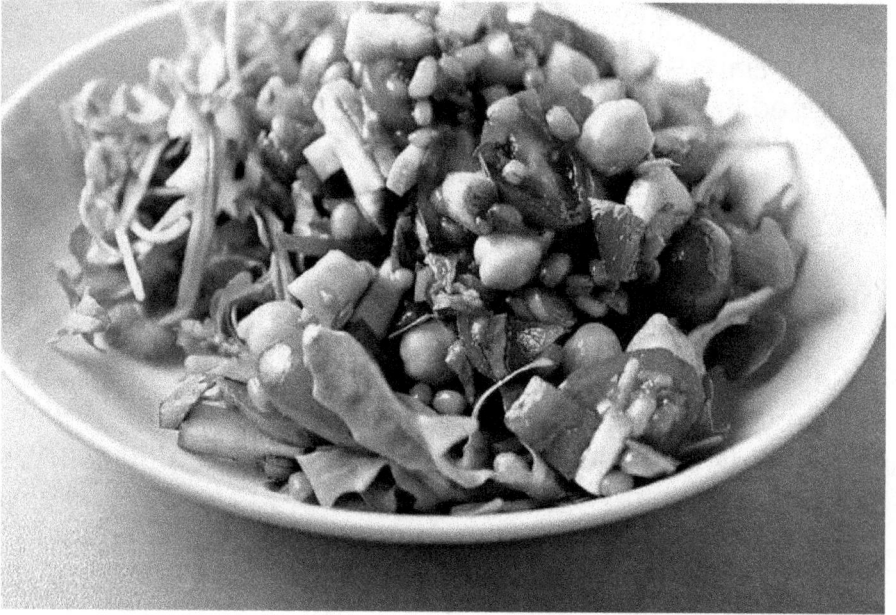

Lentil Omelet

Preparation Time: 5 minutes
Cooking Time: 10 minutes
Servings: 2

Ingredients:

8 Avocado Slices for Garnish
½ Cup Grape Tomatoes, Chopped for Garnish
½ Cup Lentils, Canned, Drained & Rinsed 1 Cup
Asparagus, Chopped
¼ Cup Onion, Chopped 1 Tablespoon Thyme
4 Eggs, Whisked

Directions:

1.Get out a bowl and whisk you egg and thyme together. Place it to the side.

2.Heat a skillet using medium heat, and cook your onion and asparagus for two to three minutes. Add in your lentils, cooking for another two minutes. It should be heated all the way through. Reduce the heat to low.

3.Get out a skillet and place it over medium heat, whisking your eggs again before adding them to the skillet. Cook for two to three minutes. They should be set on the bottom.

4.Spread your lentil and asparagus mixture on one half. Cook for another two minutes before folding the egg over the lentil filling. Cook for another two minutes.

5.Repeat with your remaining ingredients to create a second omelet.

6.Garnish with avocado before serving.

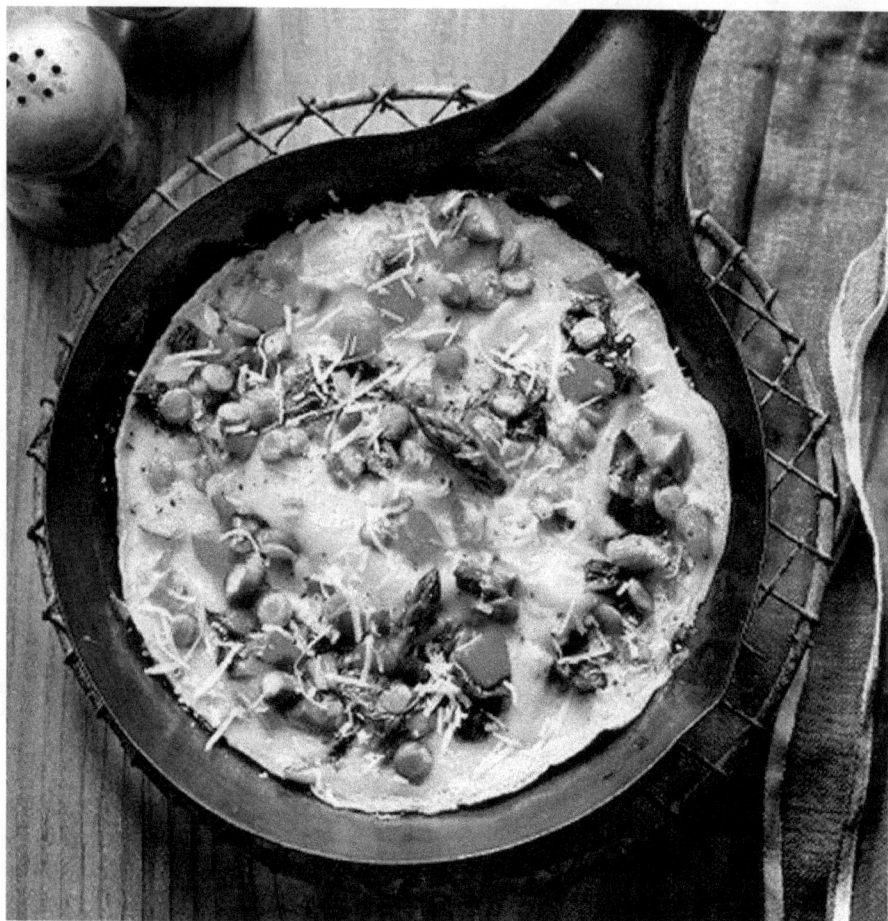

Apple Quinoa Bowl

Preparation Time: 10 minutes
Cooking Time: 15 minutes
Servings: 2

Ingredients:

½ Cup Quinoa, Uncooked
1 Cup Vanilla Almond Milk, Unsweetened
½ Teaspoon Cinnamon 2 Cinnamon Sticks Pinch Sea
Salt Toppings:
2 Tablespoons Almonds, Sliced 2 Tablespoons Hemp
Seeds
1 Cup Apple, Chopped Honey to Sweeten

Directions:

1.Rinse your quinoa using a colander and make sure it's
well drained.

2. Transfer it to a saucepan with your cinnamon,
cinnamon sticks, almond milk and salt. Bring it to a
simmer, and cover. Reduce to low, allowing it to
simmer for fifteen minutes.

3.Remove it from heat and then let it rest for five
minutes. Your almond milk should be absorbed, and you
should cook your quinoa all the way through.

4.Divide between bowls and top with your toppings.

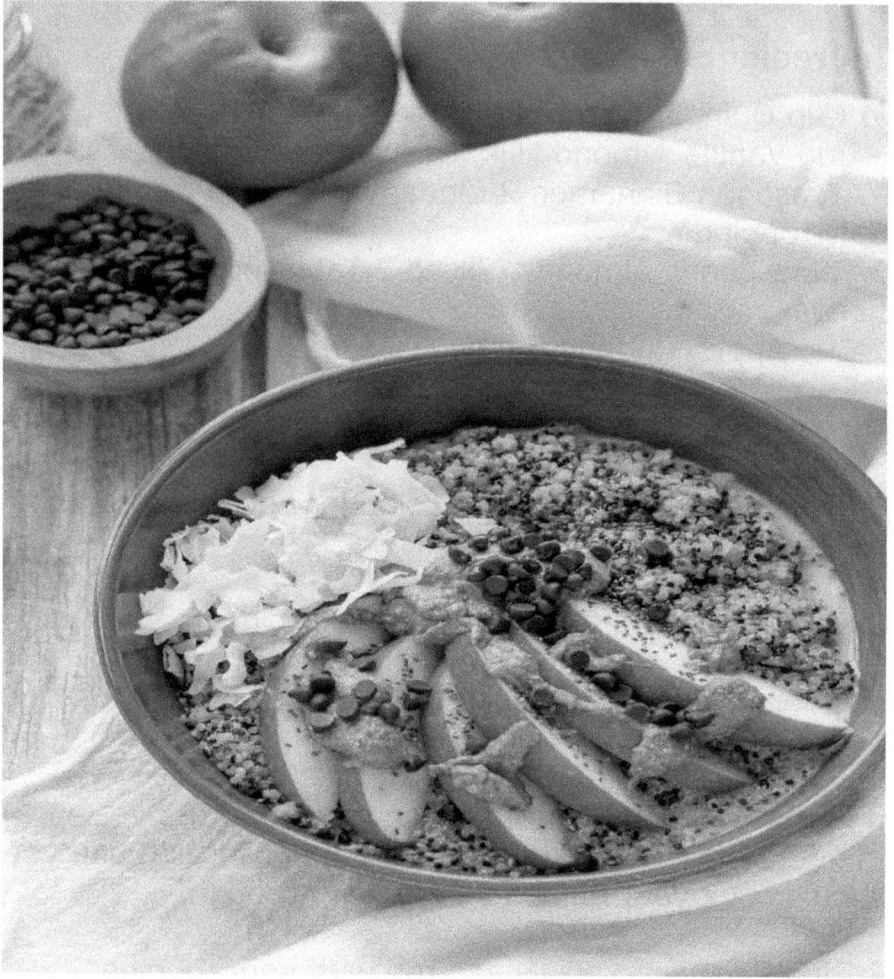

Overnight Chia Pudding

Preparation Time: 8 hours and 5 minutes
Cooking Time: 0 minutes
Servings: 2

Ingredients:
½ Cup Chia Seeds
2n Cups Coconut Milk, Light 3 Teaspoons Honey,
Divided
¼ Cup Banana, Sliced
¼ Cup Raspberries, Fresh
½ Tablespoon Almonds, Sliced
½ Tablespoon Walnuts, Chopped
2 Teaspoons Cocoa Powder, Unsweetened & Divided

Directions:

1.Mix your chia seeds, coconut milk, and two teaspoons of honey in a bowl. Portion it out into mason jars, and refrigerate for eight hours or overnight.

2.Remove them from the fridge, and top with raspberries, almonds, banana, cocoa and walnuts. Drizzle with remaining honey.

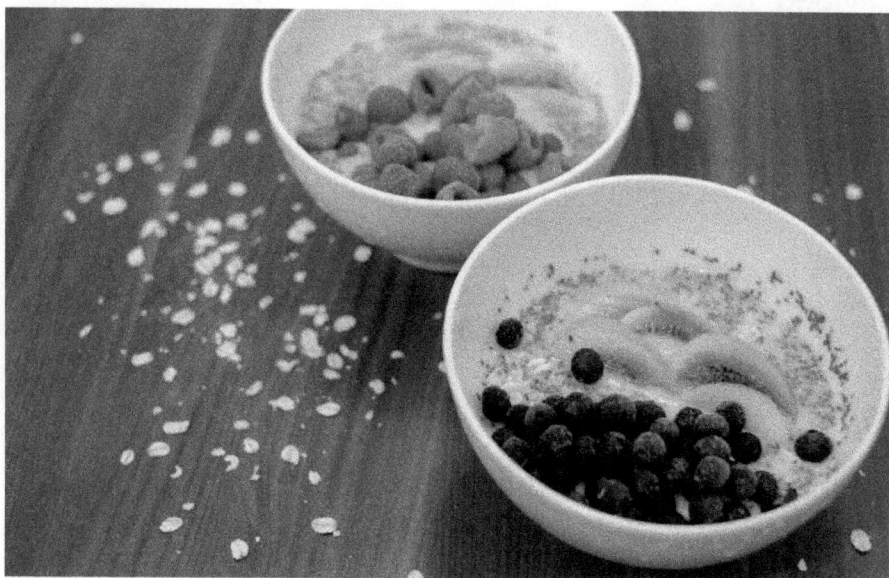

Avocado Toast

Preparation time: 10 minutes
Cooking time: 0 minutes
Servings: 2

Ingredients:

1 tablespoon goat cheese, crumbled 1 avocado, peeled, pitted and mashed A pinch of salt and black pepper
2 whole wheat bread slices, toasted
½ teaspoon lime juice
1 persimmon, thinly sliced 1 fennel bulb, thinly sliced 2 teaspoons honey
2 tablespoons pomegranate seeds

Directions:

1.In a bowl, combine the avocado with salt, pepper, lime juice and the cheese and whisk.

2.Spread this onto toasted bread slices, top each slice with the remaining ingredients and serve for breakfast.

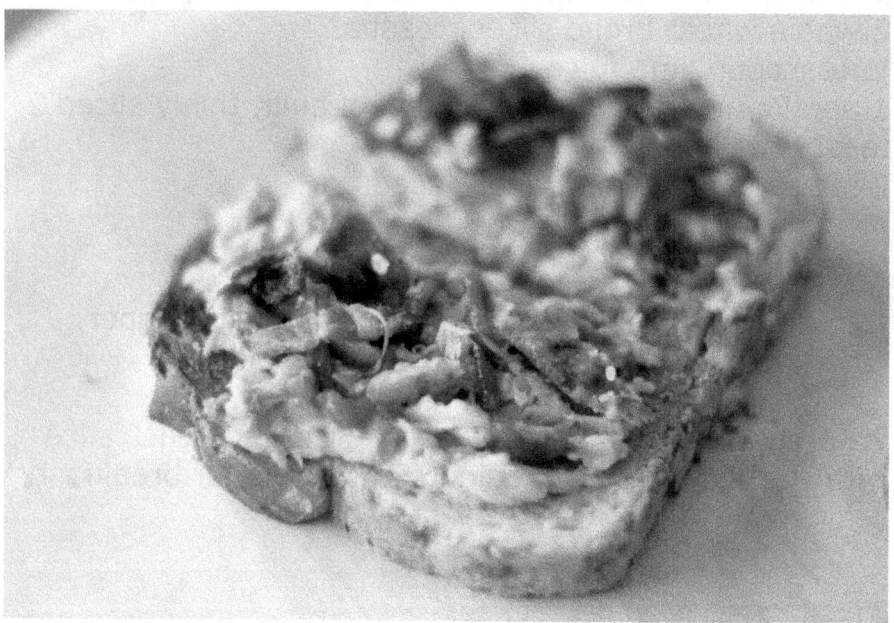

Green Juice

Preparation time: 5 minutes
Serves: 1

Ingredient:

1/4 cup fresh Italian parsley leaves
1/4 sliced pineapple
1/2 green apple
1/2 lemon
1/2 orange
A pinch of grated fresh ginger

Directions:

1. Use a juicer to run the greens cucumber parsley pineapple apple orange lemon and ginger through it pour into a large cup and serve.

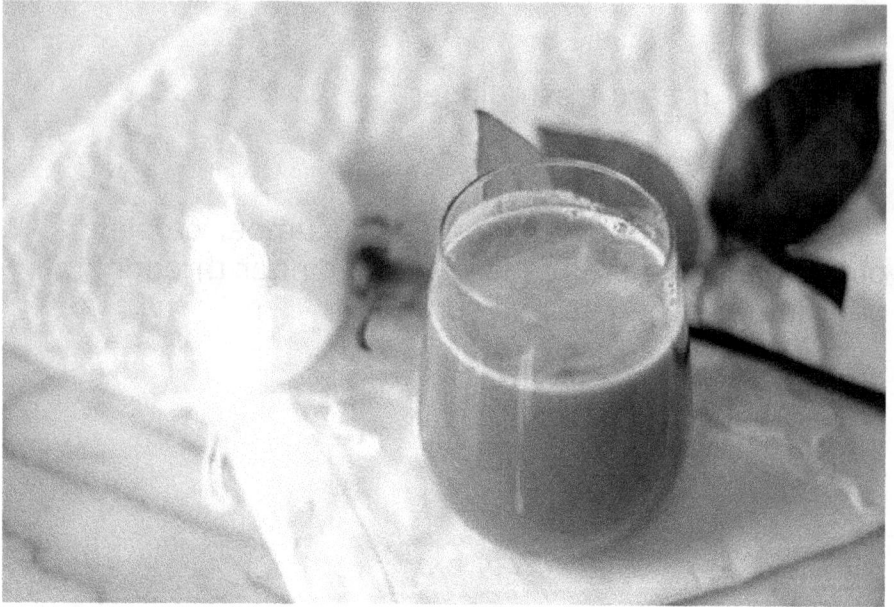

Healthy Chocolate Banana Smoothie

Preparation time: 5 minutes
Serves: 2

Ingredients:

2 bananas

4 ice cubes (if you don't have frozen banana)

1 cup unsweetened almond milk or skim milk

1 cup crushed ice

3 tablespoons unsweetened cocoa powder (to taste)

3 tablespoons sugar or honey

Directions:

1. In a blender jar pour milk and add banana almond milk ice cocoa powder and honey. Blend until smooth.

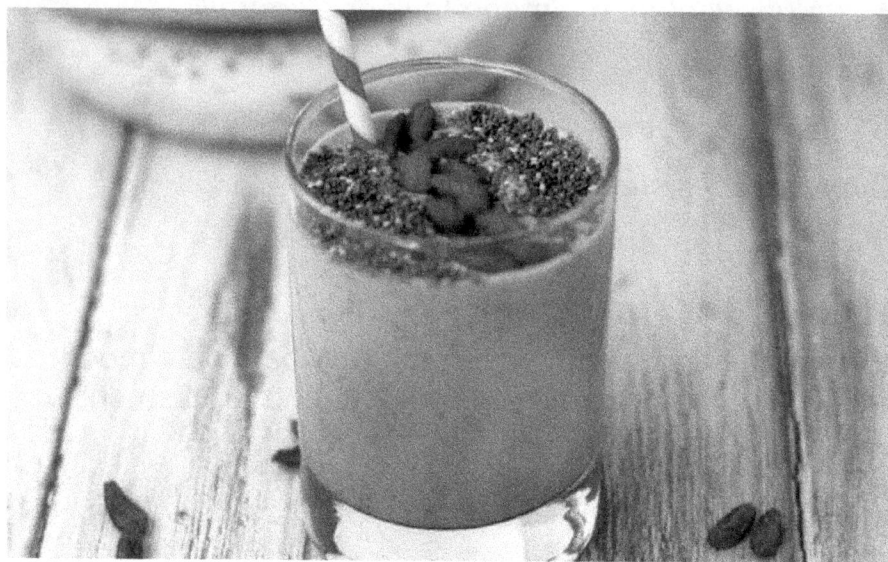

Fruit Smoothie

Preparation time: 5 minutes
Serves: 2

Ingredients:

2 cups blueberries
2 cups unsweetened almond milk
1 cup crushed ice
1/2 teaspoon ground ginger

Directions:

1. Combine the blueberries almond milk ice and ginger in a blender. Blend until smooth.

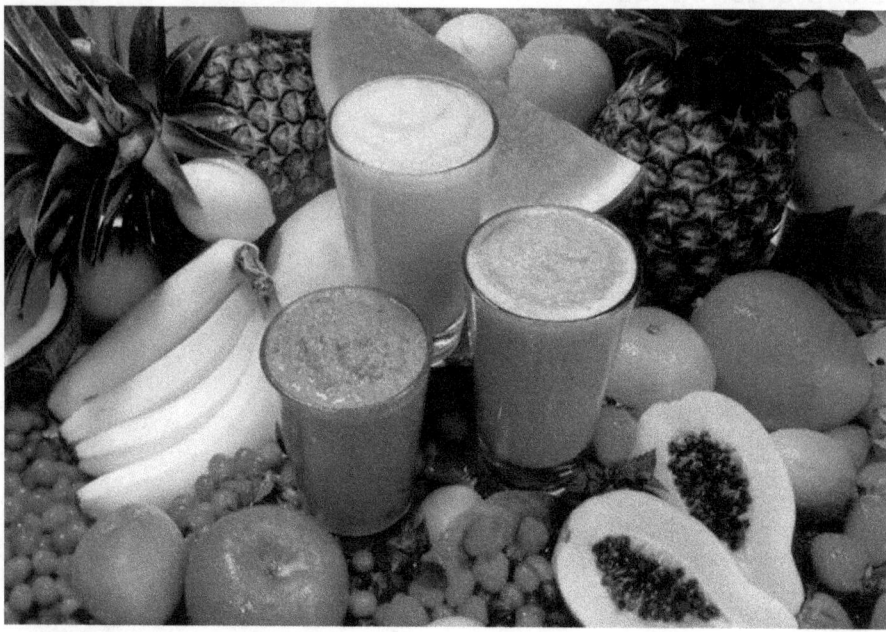

Mixed Berry and Yogurt Parfait

Preparation time: 5 minutes
Serves: 2

Ingredients:

1 cup raspberries
1 cup blackberries
1/2 cups unsweetened nonfat plain Greek yogurt
1/4 cup chopped walnuts

Directions:

1. Arrange the raspberries yogurt and blackberries in 2 bowls. Sprinkle with the walnuts.

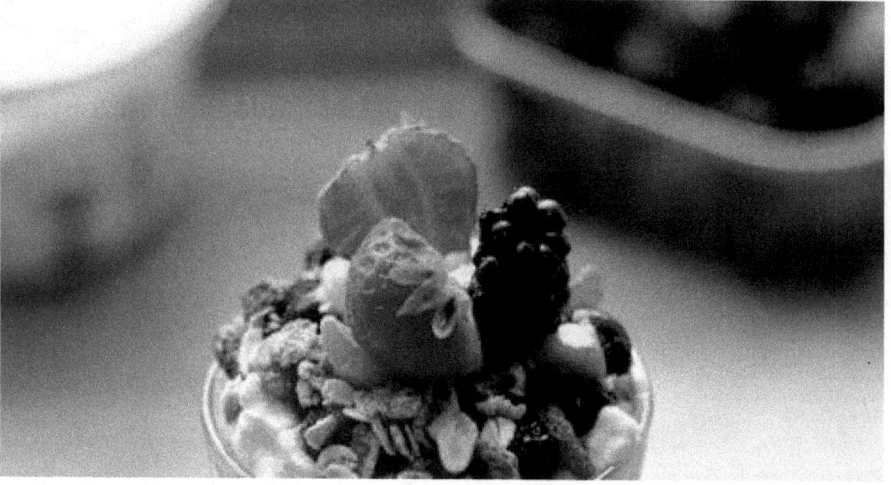

Yogurt Blueberries Honey and Mint Combination

Preparation time: 5 minutes
Serves: 2

Ingredients:

2 cups unsweetened nonfat plain Greek yogurt
1 cup blueberries
3 tablespoons honey
2 tablespoons fresh mint leaves chopped

Directions:

1. Share out the yogurt between 2 small bowls. Top with the blueberries honey and mint.

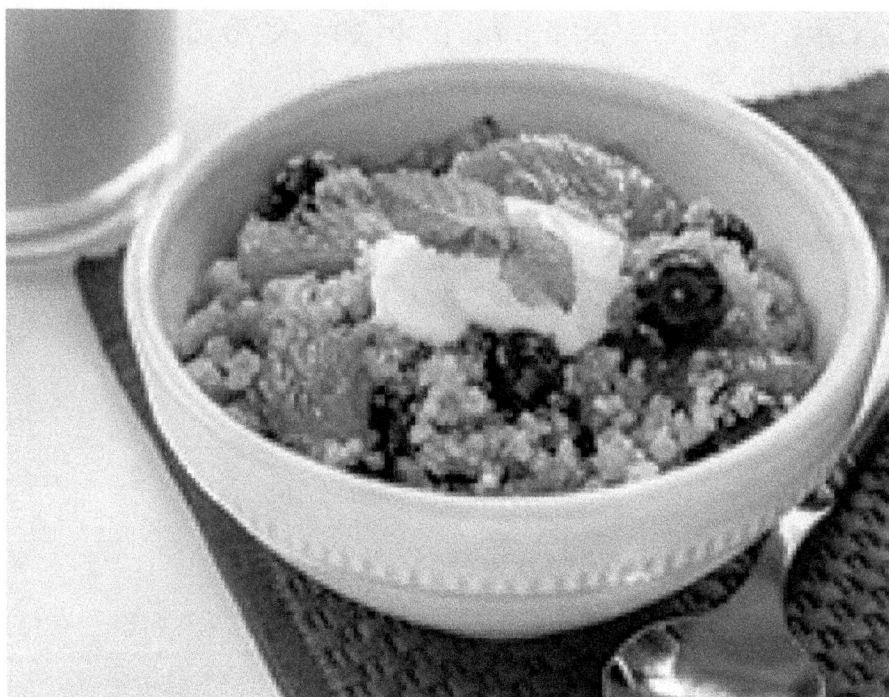

Almond and Maple Quick Grits

Preparation time: 5 minutes
Cook time: 6 minutes
Serves: 4

Ingredients:

11/2 cups water
1/2 cup unsweetened almond milk
Pinch sea salt
1/2 cup quick-cooking grits
1/2 teaspoon ground cinnamon
1/4 cup pure maple syrup
1/4 cup slivered almonds

Directions:

1.Heat the water almond milk and sea salt in a medium saucepan over medium-high heat until it boils.

2.Stirring constantly with a spoon and slowly add the grits. Continue stirring to prevent lumps and bring the mixture to a slow boil. Reduce the heat to medium-low.

3.Simmer for 6 minutes stirring frequently,continue till the water is completely absorbed.

4.Add the cinnamon syrup and almonds while you stir.

5.Cook for 1 minute more and stir.

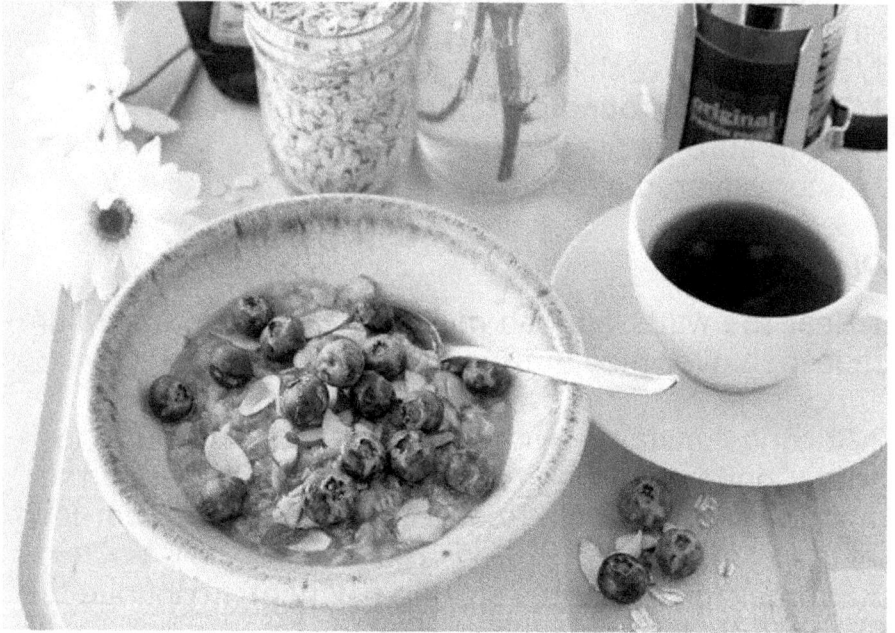

Oatmeal Topped with Berries and Sunflower Seeds

Preparation time: 15 minutes
Serves: 4

Ingredients:

13/4 cups water
1/2 clip unsweetened almond milk
1 cup old-fashioned oats
1/2 cup blueberries
1/2 cup raspberries
1/4 cup sunflower seeds
A pinch of sea salt

Directions:

1.In a saucepan over medium-high heat, then heat the almond milk and sea salt to a boil.

2.Gently pour in the oat as you stir. Reduce the heat and cook for 5 - 6 minutes.

3.Cover and let the oatmeal stand for 2 minutes more. Stir and serve topped with the blueberries raspberries and sunflower seeds.

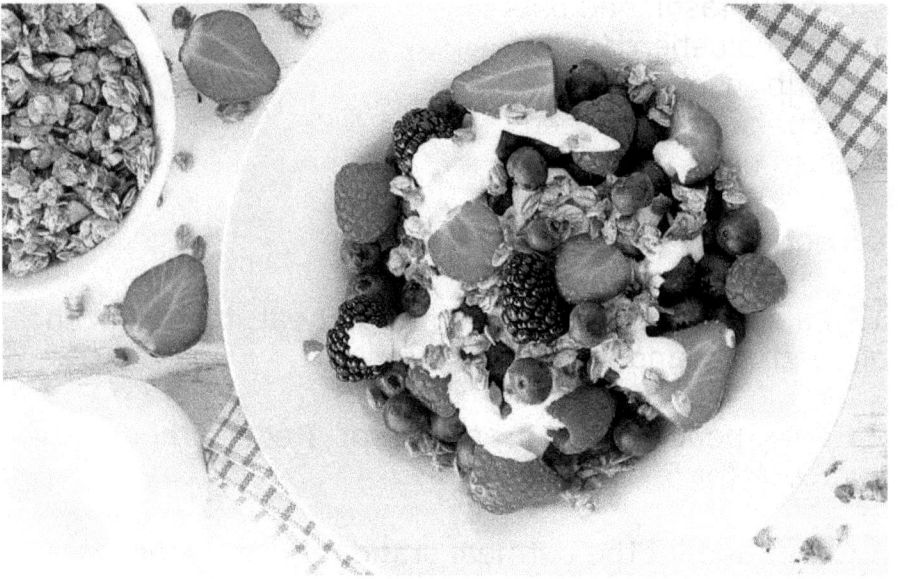

Eggy Bread

Preparation time: 30 minutes
Serves: 6

Ingredients:

6 light whole-wheat bread slices
11/2 clips unsweetened almond milk
2 eggs beaten
2 egg whites beaten
1 teaspoon vanilla extract
Zest of 1 orange
Juice of 1 orange
1 teaspoon ground nutmeg
Nonstick cooking spray

Directions:;

1.Using a shallow bowl whisk the almond milk eggs egg white vanilla orange zest and juice and nutmeg.

2.Place the bread in one single layer in a 9-by-13-inch baking dish. Pour the milk and egg mixture over the top. Allow the bread to soak for about few minutes turning once.

3.Spray a nonstick skillet with cooking spray and heat over medium-high heat. Working in batches add the bread and then cook for about 5 minutes per side until the custard sets.

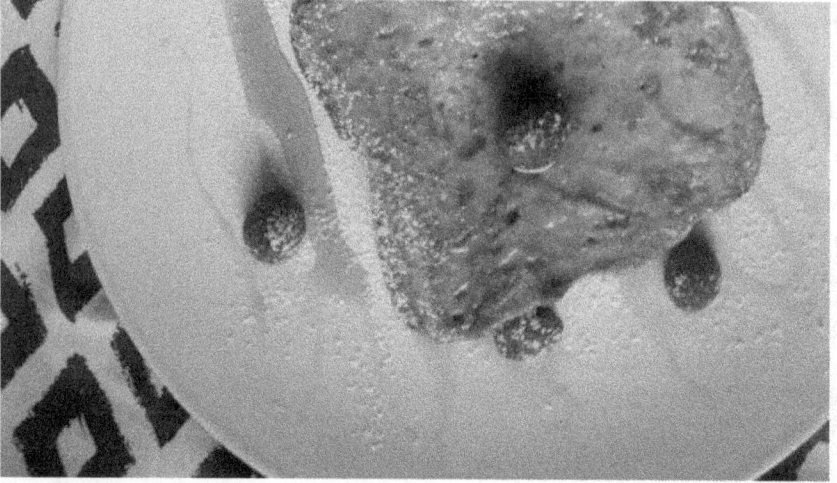

Zucchini-Tomato Frittata

Preparation time: 10 minutes
Cook time: 8 minutes
Serves: 4

Ingredients:

3 eggs
3 egg whites
1/2 cup unsweetened almond
½ milk
1/2 teaspoon sea salt
Vs teaspoon freshly ground black pepper
2 tablespoons extra-virgin olive oil
1 zucchini chopped
8 cherry tomatoes halved
1/4 cup (about 2 ounces) grated Parmesan cheese

Directions:

1.Preheat the oven's broiler to high temperature of about 400'F adjusting the oven rack to the center position.

2.Vigorously whisk the eggs egg whites almond milk sea salt and pepper in a shallow bowel. Set aside.

3.In an about 12-inch ovenproof skillet heat the olive oil until it shimmers.

4.Now add the zucchini and tomatoes and cook for 5 minutes stirring occasionally.

5.Pour the egg cream over the vegetables and cook for about 4 minutes without stirring until the eggs set around the edges.

6.Using a silicone spatula pull the set eggs away from the edges of the pan. Tilt the pan in all Directions:s to allow the unset eggs to fill the spaces along the edges. Cook for about 4 minutes more without stirring until the edges set again.

7.Apply the eggs with the Parmesan. Transfer the pan to the broiler. Cook until the cheese melts and your eggs are puffy about 3 to 5 minutes. Cut into wedges to serve.

Scramble Egg with Smoked Salmon

Preparation time: 5 minutes
Cook time: 10 minutes
Serves: 4

Ingredients:

4 eggs
6 egg whites
1/8 teaspoon freshly ground black pepper
2 tablespoons extra-virgin olive
oil
1/2 red onion finely chopped and 4 ounces smoked salmon flaked
2 tablespoons capers drained

Directions:

1.In a small bowl whisk the eggs whites and pepper. Set aside.

2.In a large nonstick skillet heat the olive oil until it shimmers.

3.Add the onion and let cook for about 3 minutes while stirring until soft.

4.Cook the salmon and capers together for 1 minute.

5.Cook the egg mixture in a pan for about 3 to 5 minutes stirring frequently or until the eggs are set.

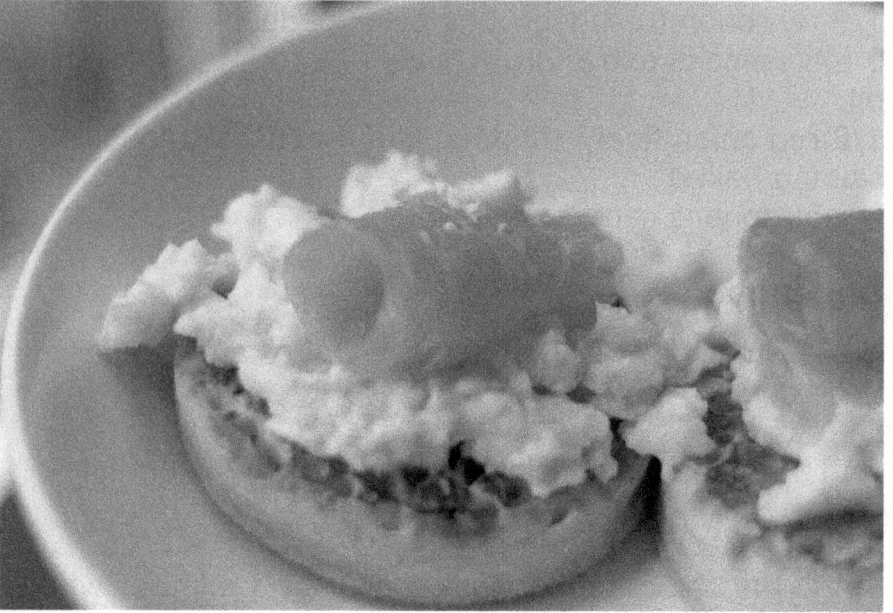

Poached Eggs with Avocado Toast

Preparation time: 10 minutes
Cook time: 5 minutes
Serves: 4

Ingredients:

2 avocados peeled and pitted
1/4 cup chopped fresh basil leaves
3 tablespoons red swine vinegar divided
Juice of 1 lemon
Zest of 1 lemon
1 garlic clove minced
1 teaspoon sea salt divided
1/8 teaspoon freshly ground black pepper
Pinch cayenne pepper plus more as needed
4 eggs

Directions:

1.In a blender combine the avocados basil 2 tablespoons of vinegar the lemon juice and zest garlic 1/2 teaspoon of sea salt pepper and cayenne. Purée for about 1 minute until smooth.

2.Fill a 12-inch nonstick skillet about three-fourths full of water and place it over medium heat. Add the residual tablespoon of vinegar and the remaining 1/2 teaspoon of sea salt. Bring the water to a simmer.

3.Carefully crack the eggs into custard cups. Holding the cups just barely above the water carefully slip theeggs into the simmering water one at a time.

4.Turn off the heat and then cover the skillet. Let the eggs sit for 5 minutes without agitating the pan or removing the lid.

5.Using a slotted spoon carefully lift the eggs from the water allowing them to drain completely. Place each egg on a plate and spoon the avocado purée over the top.

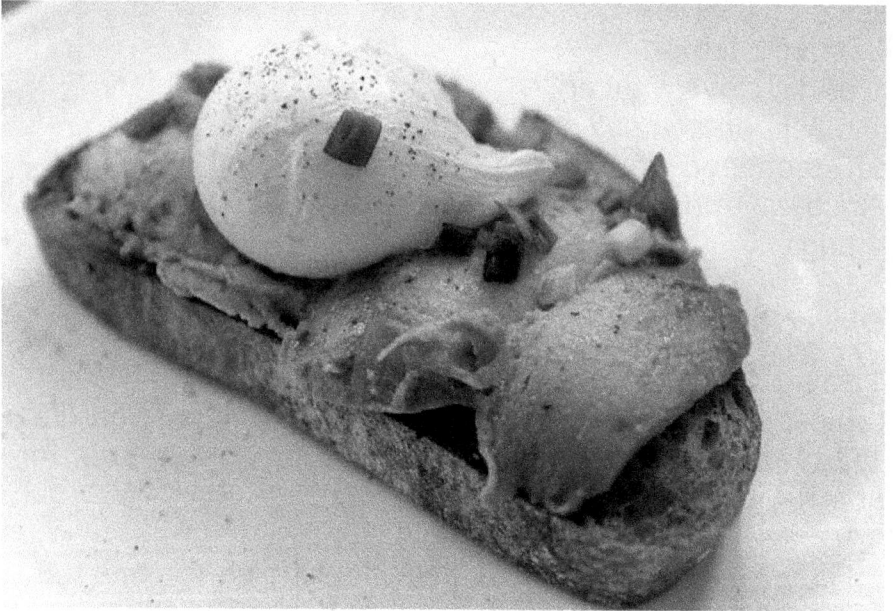

Poached Pears

Preparation Time: 15 minutes
Cooking Time: 30 minutes
Servings: 4

Ingredients:

4 Pears, Whole
¼ Cup Apple Juice 1 Cup Orange Juice
1 Teaspoon Cinnamon
1 Teaspoon Nutmeg
½ Cup Raspberries, Fresh 2 Tablespoons Orange Zest

Directions:

1.Combine your apple juice, orange juice, nutmeg and cinnamon in a bowl. Peel your pears and make sure to leave the stems on.

2.Remove the core, but make sure to remove them from the bottom.
Combine your juices and pears in a shallow pan. Cook over medium heat, and bring it to a simmer.

3.Allow it to simmer for a half hour.

4.Turn them regularly, making sure they don't come to a boil. Garnish with orange zest and raspberries.

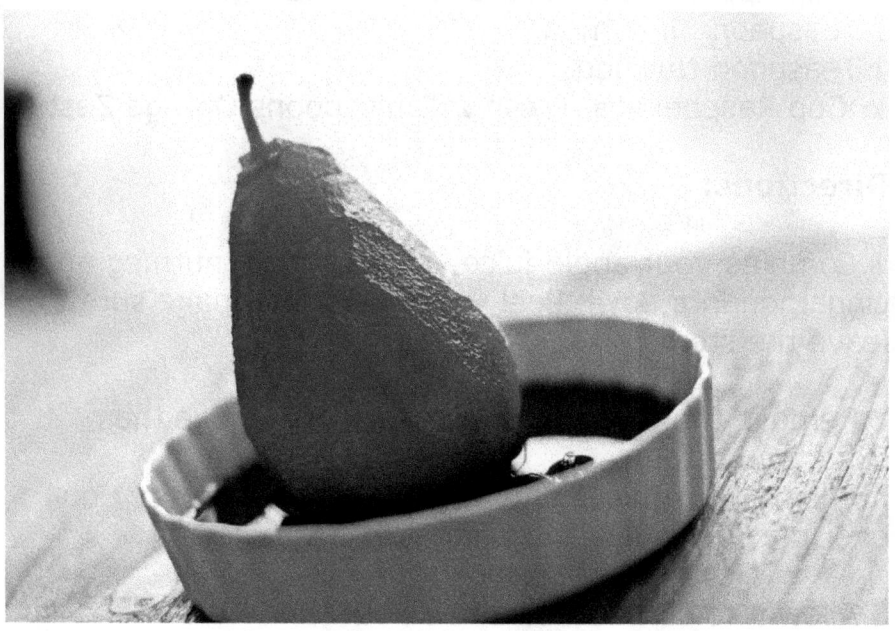

Marinated Berries

Preparation Time: 2 hours and 15 minutes
Cooking Time: 0 minutes
Servings: 2

Ingredients:
¼ Cup Balsamic Vinegar
½ Cup Strawberries
½ Cup Blueberries
½ Cup Raspberries
2 Shortbread Biscuits
2 Tablespoons Brown Sugar and 1 Teaspoon Vanilla
Extract, Pure

Directions:

1.Start by mixing your brown sugar, vanilla and balsamic vinegar in a bowl, and then blend your berries in another bowl. Pour your marinade on top of the fruit, and allow it to marinate for ten to fifteen minutes.

2.Drain, and then allow it to chill for up to two hours.

3.Distribute the chilled fruit in bowls served with shortbread on the side.

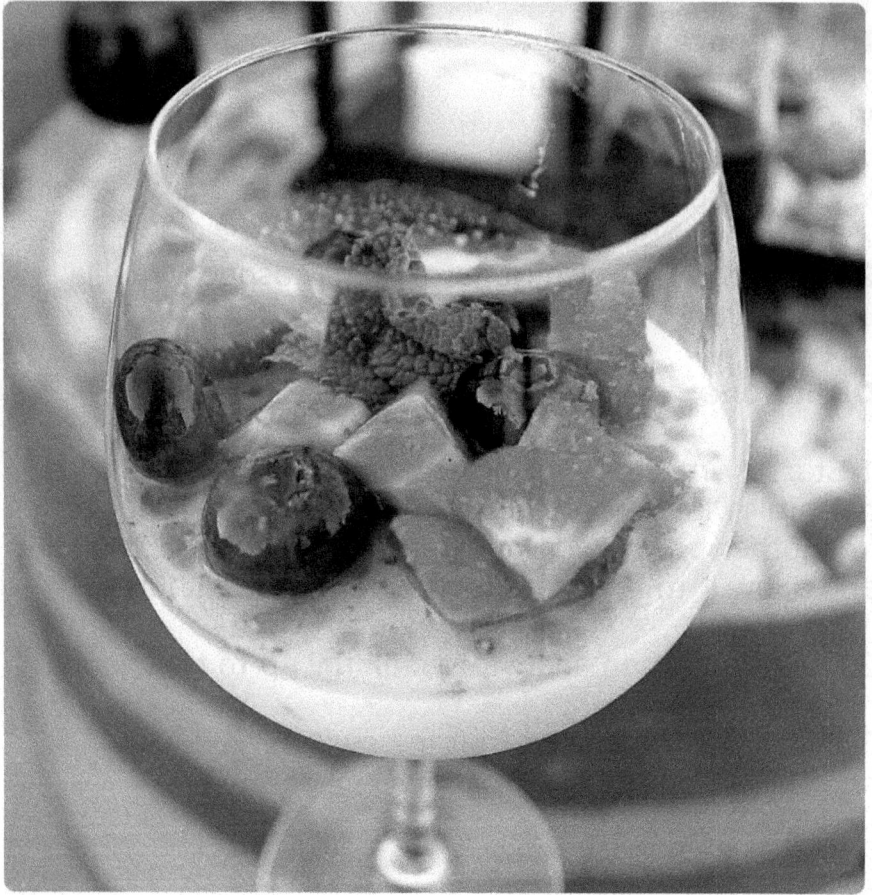

Cannellini Bean Soup

Preparation time: 5 minutes
Cooking time: 20 minutes
Servings: 4

Ingredients:

Two sliced potatoes
2 cups vegetable broth
Two cans of cannellini beans 1-2 diced garlic cloves
1/8 tsp pepper and 1/3 cup white wine
1/2 tsp paprika 1/2 tsp salt
1 tbsp tomato paste
1 tbsp of olive oil
One sprig rosemary
One diced onion
One diced carrot
1 cup spinach
One diced celery stalk

Directions:

1.Heat the oil in a big kettle. Add the diced celery, carrot, and onion until the oil shimmers. Cook for 5 minutes, stirring until the onion is soft and turns translucent.

2.Add the potatoes, tomato paste, beans, garlic, rosemary (whatever is better for you, the whole sprig, sliced, or dried), and paprika. (if you use it). (if you use it). (if you use it). (if you use it). (if you use it). (if you use it). Cook for about 1 minute, stirring constantly.

3.Pour in the wine, mix well, and let it boil for another minute until it has evaporated.

4.Then include frozen spinach in the vegetables' broth and a pleasant pinch of salt & pepper. Boost the heat, boil the mixture, gently cover the kettle, and reduce the heat and simmer for 15 minutes.

5.Remove the pot from the heat until the potatoes are soft and the soup is dense and fluffy, then remove the rosemary sprig*. Taste and season with pepper and salt. Based on the vegetable broth or your preferences, you can need more salt.

6.Break into cups, drizzle with extra virgin olive oil or olive oil, and add more ground black pepper as you prefer. Serve with the crusty whole-grain bread, and add fresh parmesan cheese for extra spice if you do not keep it vegan. Enjoy! Enjoy!

Garlic, sweet potato, and chickpea soup

Preparation time: 10 minutes
Cooking time: 30 minutes
Servings: 4-6

Ingredients:
Lemon juice
Eight cloves garlic, sliced
400 g chickpeas
350 g cooked sweet potato
30 g olive oil
2 tsp ground turmeric
2 tsp dried thyme
1 tsp salt
One chopped onion
½ tsp cayenne pepper

Directions:

1.In a big saucepan with water, place the garlic, olive oil, and onions: this produces more steam to rapidly tender the garlic. Then bring the fire to a boil and simmer for five min until the water evaporates and the garlic is very tender.

2.Add the sweet potatoes, salt, thyme, turmeric, chickpeas, cayenne, and 800 ml of water, and bring to a boil until the sweet potatoes have further softened. Remove from the sun and slightly cool off.

3.In a mixer, puree the mixture until creamy. If necessary, return to the pan, change the consistency

with additional water, and then heat it until it boils.
Divide between 4 and 6 bowls and apply a drizzle

4.of lemon juice and a few shreds of black pepper to
each bowl.

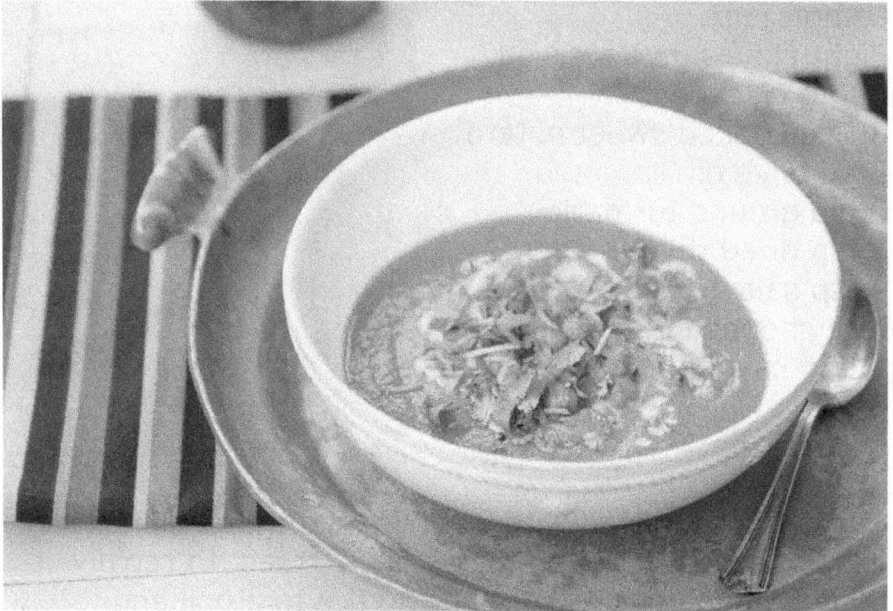

Kumara, coconut, and lemongrass soup

Preparation time: 10 minutes
Cooking time: 25 minutes
Servings: 6

Ingredients:

One chopper White onion
5 cups of Vegetable Stock Thai Basil - for garnish
2 lb chopped Sweet Potatoes
2 tbsp Olive Oil
2 Lemongrass Stalks 2 Kaffir Lime Leaves
½ tsp chopped ginger
½ tbsp Chopped garlic
½ cup Coconut Milk
Four chopped Celery Stalks

Directions:

1.On a moderate flame, heat the olive oil. Sweat until the onion is transparent, the chopped onion, ginger, lemongrass, garlic, lime leaves, and celery.

2.Add in the vegetable supply and sweet potatoes. Carry to a boil, reduce the heat until it is cooked and then simmer cover for around 25 min or until the sweet potatoes are softened.

3.Now give a minute for the soup to cool off. Please cut the lime leaves and the lemongrass before you mix it into a smooth broth. Move all the ingredients carefully into your blender or cream the soup with a handheld blender.

4.Put the soup back in a clean dish, reheat, and add the milk from the coconut. Taste the broth and season with white pepper and some salt, if possible.

5.Reheat the soup before eating, put it in bowls, and spread some Thai basil on top.

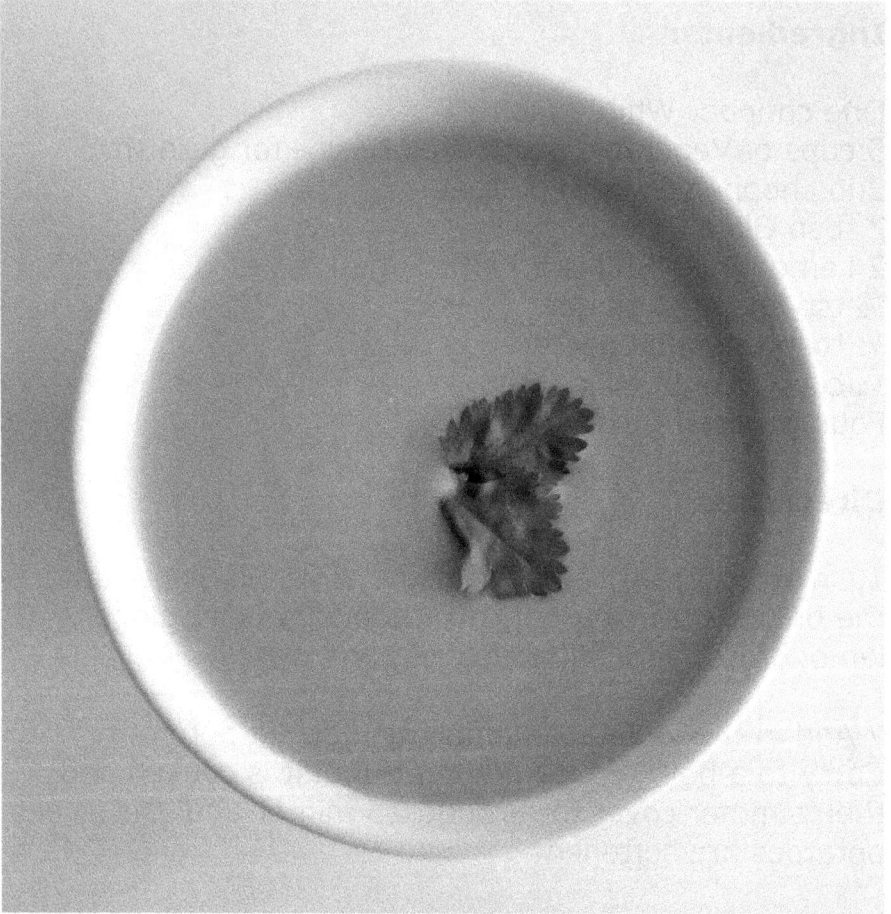

Moroccan Chickpea Soup

Preparation time: 15 minutes
Cooking time: 30 minutes
Servings: 3

Ingredients:
coriander sprigs
500 ml of vegetable stock
40 g seed mix, roasted
410 g tin chickpeas
400 g chopped tomatoes
1 tsp cumin seeds
1 tbsp olive oil
One chopped red pepper
One chopped onion
One crushed garlic clove One chopped carrot

Directions:

1.Heat the olive oil in a saucepan, then add the seeds of onion, carrot, garlic, pepper, and cumin and fry for around 5 minutes. Stir in the stock and the tomatoes, and cook for 5 minutes.

2.Using a hand blender to purée the onions, stir in chickpeas, and heat them for 2 minutes.

3.Adorn with coriander/beans. With bread, serve.

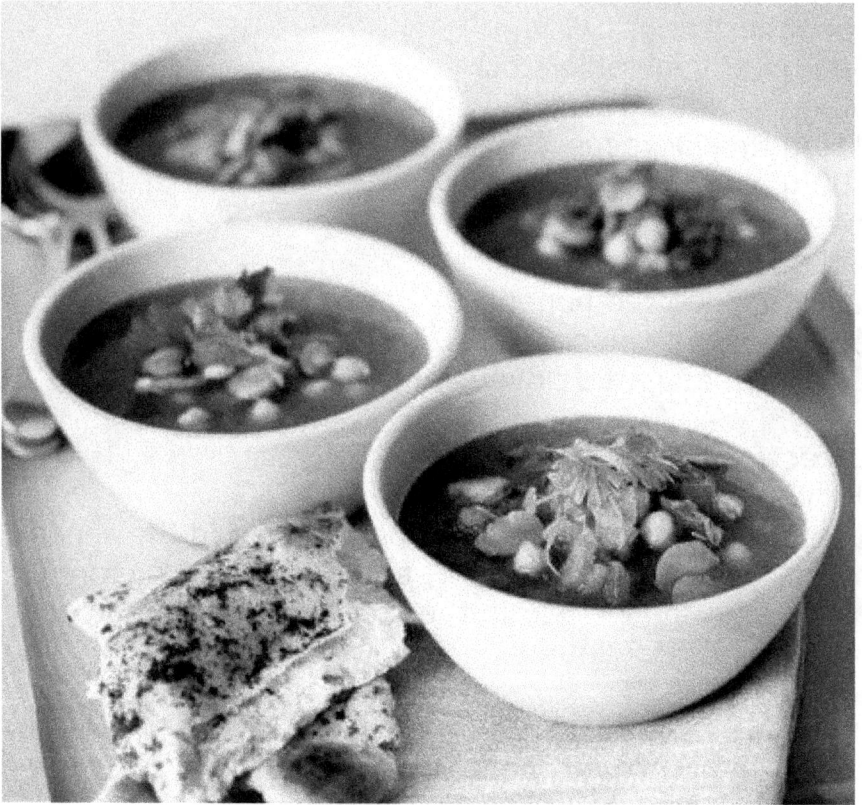

Ribollita

Preparation time: 15 minutes
Cooking time: 25 minutes
Servings: 10

Ingredients:

1 1/2 tsp salt
14 oz crushed tomatoes
One red onion, chopped
1 lb chopped cavolo nero
1/2 lb loaf of bread
Two chopped carrots
Three cloves garlic, chopped
3 tbsp olive oil
Four celery stalks, chopped
4 cups white beans, cooked chopped black olives
1/2 tsp of red pepper flakes zest of one lemon

Directions:

1.Mix the olive oil, garlic, carrot, celery, and red onion in the largest dense pot over medium heat. Sweat the vegetables for 10 -15 minutes, but stop further browning. Add the tomatoes and flakes of red pepper and cook for another ten minutes, long enough to make the tomatoes thicken a little. Add the cavolo nero, and 8 cups of water, 3 cups of beans, per 2 liters. Bring it to a boil, reduce the heat and cook for around 15 minutes until the greens are tender.

2.Meanwhile, with a generous splash of water, mash or puree the remaining beans - till smooth. Tear the bread into chunks. Add the bread and the beans to the soup. Simmer, stirring regularly, for 20 minutes or so, before

the bread disintegrates and the soup becomes thick.
Add the salt, taste and if appropriate, add more. Stir in
the zest of the lemon.

3.Serve instantly, or cool overnight and refrigerate.
With a bit of olive oil and some chopped olives, finish
each serving.

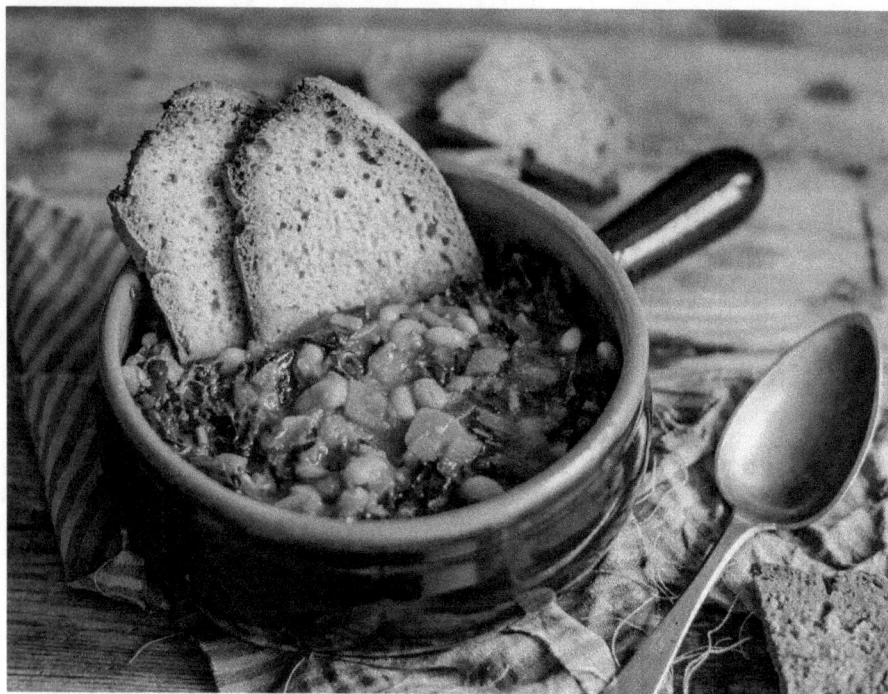

Broccoli soup

Preparation time: 10 minutes
Cooking time: 25 minutes
Servings: 6

Ingredients:
One onion, chopped
One stalk celery, chopped
2 cups of milk
3 cups chicken brot
3 tbsp all-purpose flour and 5 tbsp butter
8 cups broccoli florets black pepper to taste

Directions:

1.In a medium-sized stock container, heat two tablespoons of butter and sauté the celery and onion until tender. Add the broccoli and broth, then cover for 10 minutes and simmer.
2.In a mixer, pour the broth, filling the pitcher but no more than halfway full. With the folded kitchen towel, keep the blender's lid down and start the blender carefully, using a few short pulses to transfer the soup before leaving it to puree. Purée until smooth and dump into a clean pot in batches. Alternately, right in the frying pot, you should use a stick blender to puree the broth.
3.Melt three tablespoons of butter in a shallow saucepan, whisk in the flour and add the cream. Stir until bubbly and thick, and apply to the broth. Season and eat with pepper.

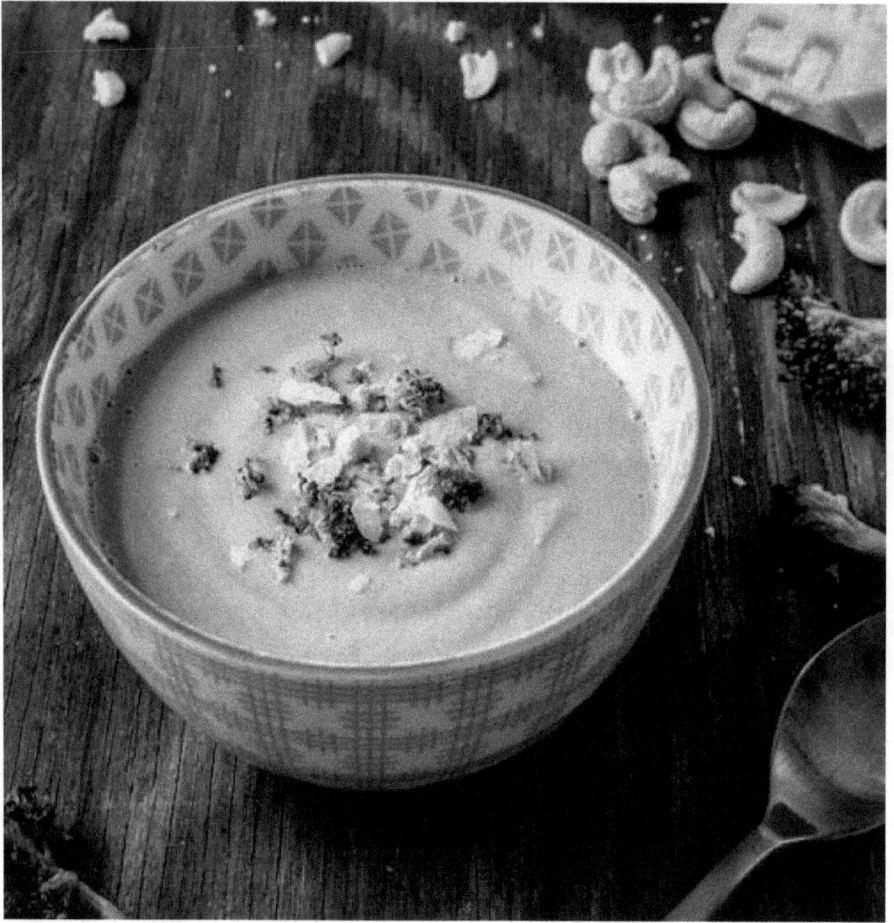

Mushroom soup

Preparation time: 5 minutes
Cooking time: 45 minutes
Servings: 6

Ingredients:
Salt to taste
Black pepper to taste Six sprigs thyme
4 cups chicken stock 3 tbsp olive oil
1/4 cup whipping cream
1/4 cup Cognac
1/4 cup chopped chives
1/2 cup minced shallot One sprig rosemary
1 lb mixed mushrooms
1 lb cremini mushrooms

Directions:

1.Chop the mushroom stems roughly and let them simmer
and covered for about an hour in the chicken broth.

2. In a large skillet, heat the oil and sauté each shallot until they are transparent. Lightly add the spices, salt, and pepper.

3.Chop the mushroom caps beautifully and precisely into the 1/2-inch dice. Add them as they are sliced into the shallots. Keep the heat very low until the mushroom fluid is released and then reabsorbed, and cook gently. Shake the cup so that they do not stick. Remove the rosemary and thyme.

4.Turn the heat up, then add the Cognac. Flame it up if you just feel like Chef-y. Cook down the mushroom cap or shallot mixture until well-reduced and begin to turn the edges a bit golden.

5.Strain the fungus from the broth of the chicken.

6.To the filtered broth, apply the wonderful shallot mixture and mushroom cap and heat it gently.

7.Swirl in and serve the cream and chives. Or serve, if you like to get fancy, in tiny sipping bowls topped with chives and softly whipped cream.

Chickpea & Pomegranate Dip

Preparation time: 10 minutes
Cooking time: 0 minute
Servings: 5

Ingredients:

3 tbsp pomegranate molasses
2 tbsp chopped mint
2 tbsp chopped coriander
12 oz chickpeas
1/4 cup of red Onion
1/4 cup crumbled feta cheese 1/2 tsp salt
1/2 tsp hot pepper flakes
1/2 cup olive oil
One clove garlic minced 1 tsp ground cumin

Directions:

1.Put pulse chickpeas, pomegranate molasses, oil, all but one teaspoon (about 5 mL) both of the mint & coriander along with cumin, salt, and pepper flakes together in the food processor until mixed, but still a little bit chunky.

2.Onion pulse; whisk in garlic. Scrap the serving bowl into it. (Make- ahead: Up to 24 hours to cover and refrigerate.) Dust with feta and leftover mint and coriander.

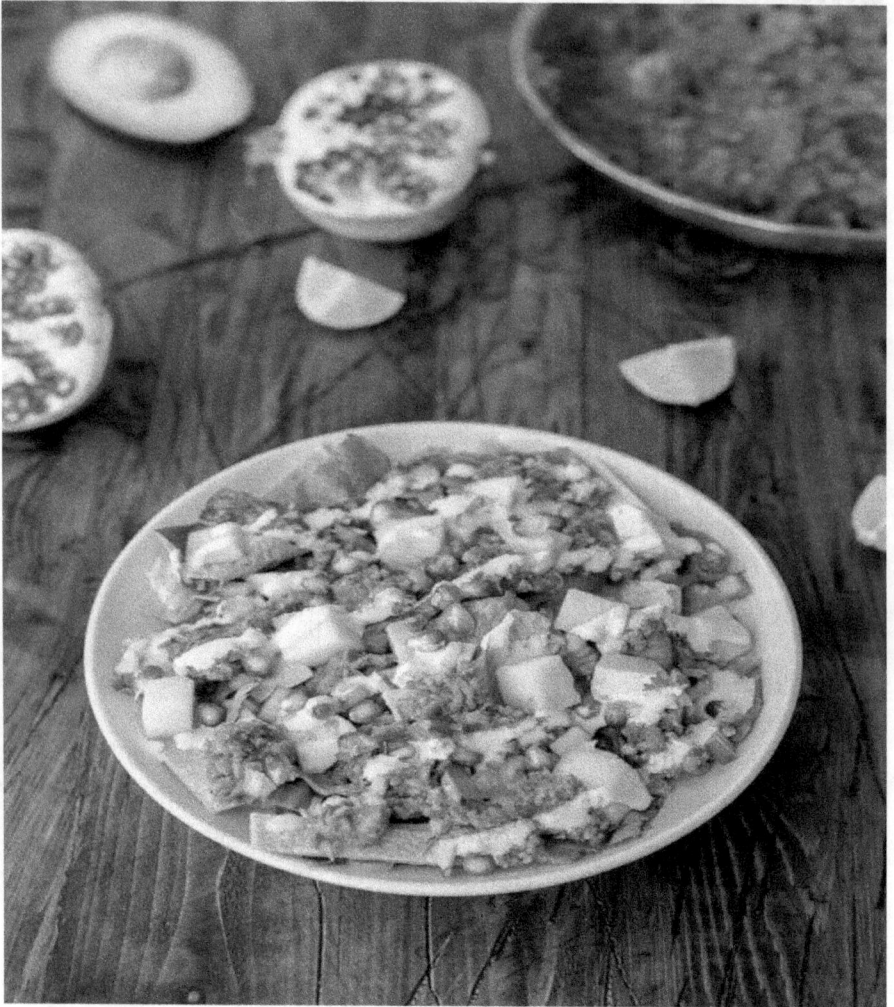

Mushroom & Cardamom, Squash Soup

Preparation time: 8 minutes
Cooking time: 30 minutes
Servings: 3

Ingredients:

1 tsp ginger One leek
1 tsp Celtic sea salt
125 ml of coconut cream
200 g mushrooms
250 ml passata
300 ml of water
350g of peeled squash Four cardamom pods 1 cup herbs
Dash of coconut oil

Directions:

1.In a bowl, sugar, milk, salt, ginger, and past, cardamom into a squash. Cook and for 15 minutes.

2.Blend the mixture.

3.Sauté mushrooms in heated oil for five minutes.

4.Serve in serving dish by making layers and serve.

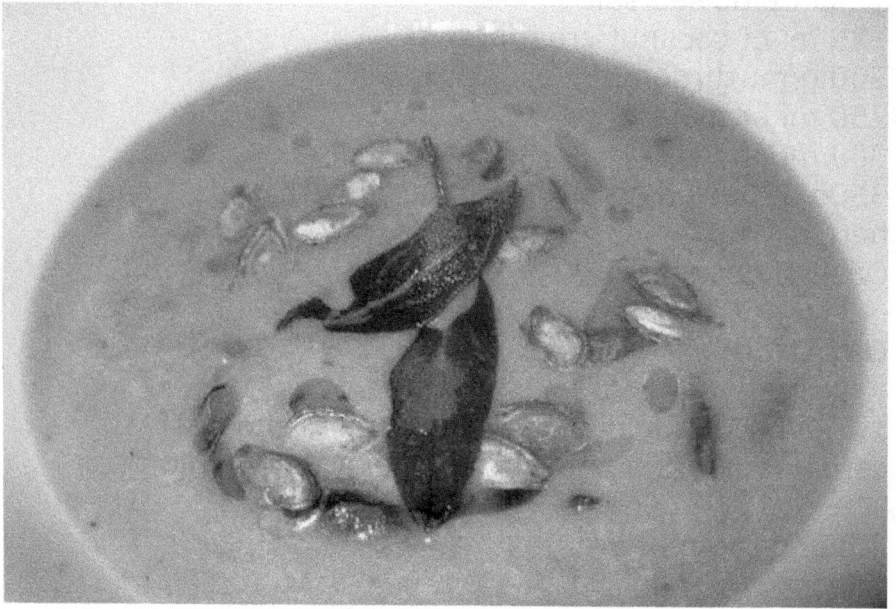

Pomegranate Avocado Salsa

Preparation time: 10 minutes
Cooking time: 10 minutes
Servings: 6

Ingredients:

1/3 cup red onion diced
1/3 cup chopped cilantro
Two pomegranates sliced One jalapeno chopped
One avocado
The juice of 1 lime and 1 tsp sea salt

Directions:

1. Mix all the ingredients and serve.

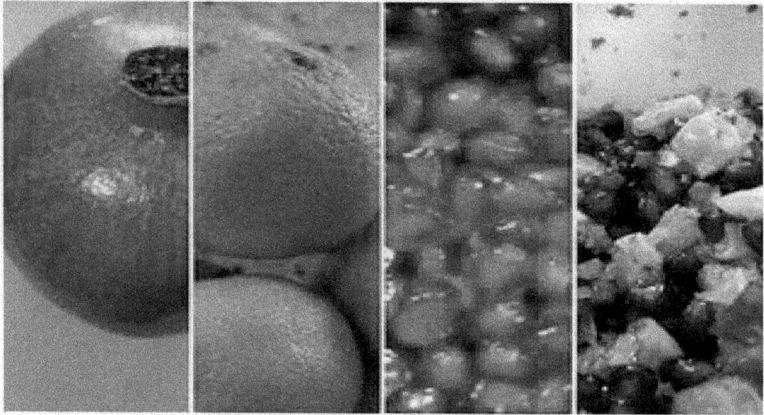

White Bean Bruschetta

Preparation time: 5 minutes
Cooking time: 10minutes
Servings: 6

Ingredients:
1 -2 clove garlic sliced
1 cup cannellini beans, cooked
½ tsp red pepper flakes
2 tbsp balsamic vinegar and 2 tbsp olive oil
2 tbsp basil leaves
6 slices Italian bread
Garlic
Salt to taste Pepper to taste

Directions:

1.Mix all the items in a jar except bread.

2.Toast the bread and spread the mixture, and serve.

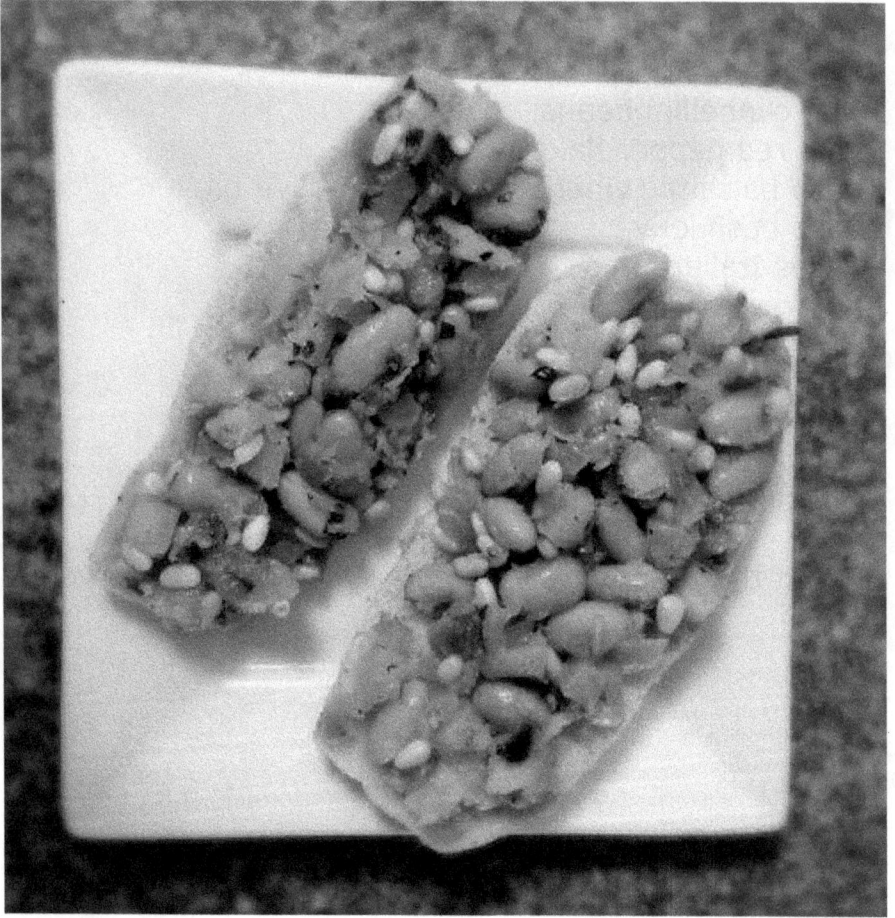

Baked Fish Fillets

Preparation time: 10 minutes
Cooking time: 20 minutes
Servings: 6

Ingredients:

2 tbsp lemon juice
2 lb mackerel fillets
1 tsp salt
1 tbsp vegetable oil
¼ cup butter, melted
⅛ tsp paprika
⅛ tsp black pepper

Directions:

1.Mix all the items in a bowl except fillets.

2.Coat fillets with the mixture and bake in a preheated oven at 350 degrees for 25 minutes.

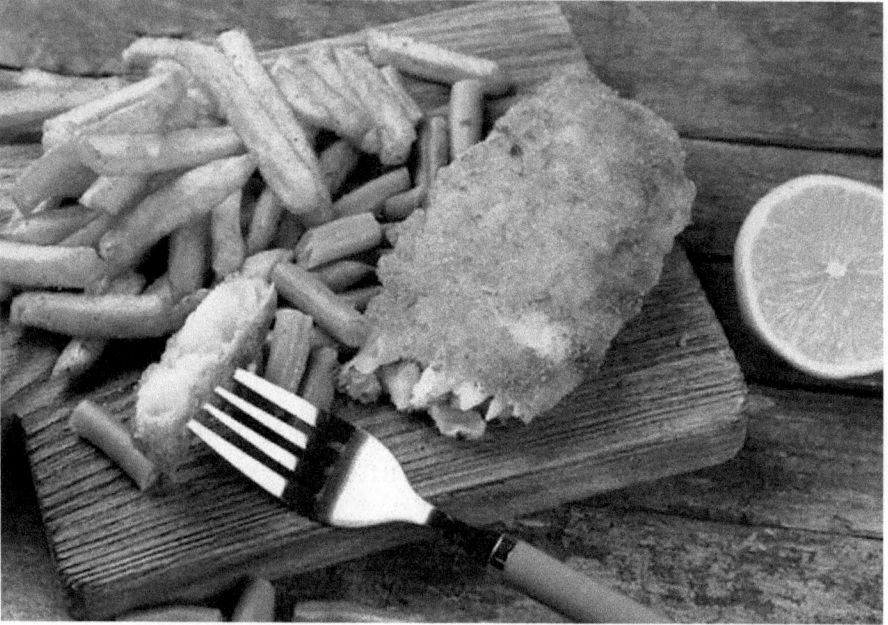

Black Bean-Salmon Stir-Fry

Preparation time: 5 minutes
Cooking time: 20 minutes
Servings: 4

Ingredients:

2 tsp cornstarch
2 tbsp rice vinegar
2 tbsp sauce black bean garlic 12 oz mung bean sprouts
1 tbsp canola oil 1 tbsp rice wine 1 lb salmon
One pinch of red pepper
1 cup diced scallions
¼ cup of water

Directions:

1.Mix all the ingredients except salmon and set aside. The sauce is ready.

2.Cook salmon in heated oil for three minutes from each side.

3.Add the sauce to salmon and cook for a minute.

4.Mix in scallions and beans and cook for five minutes.

Michael Symon's Grilled Salmon and Zucchini Salad

Preparation time: 8 minutes
Cooking time: 8 minutes
Servings: 4

Ingredients:

¼ cup chopped fresh dill
¼ cup sliced almonds, toasted
½ tsp black pepper, divided
¾ tsp kosher salt, divided One lemon
3 cups sliced zucchini
3 tbsp olive oil, divided
24 oz salmon fillets

Directions:

1.Coat fillets with salt, pepper, and oil and grill over a preheated grill for five minutes for each side. Transfer in a plate.

2.Mix all the remaining ingredients and pour over fillets.

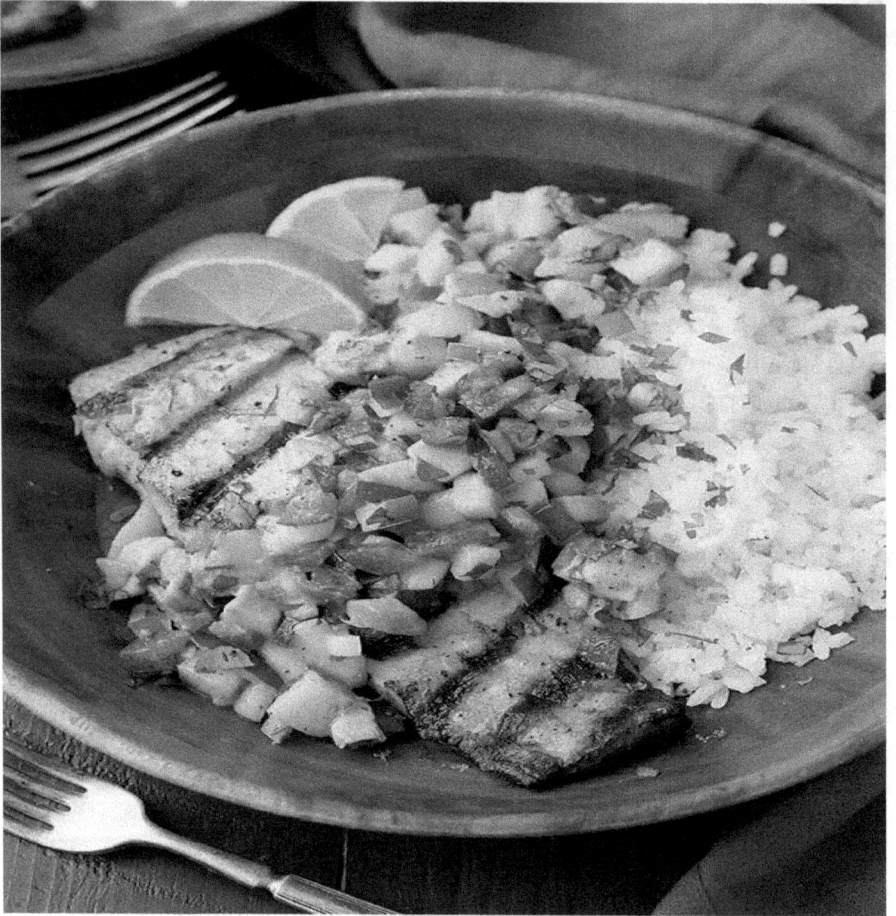

Grilled Salmon with Mustard & Herbs

Preparation time: 5 minutes
Cooking time: 40 minutes
Servings: 4

Ingredients:

¼ tsp salt
One clove garlic 1 lb salmon
1 tbsp Dijon mustard
Two lemons sliced
30 sprigs mixed herbs

Directions:

1.Arrange a layer of lemon followed by herbs on a baking tray.

2. Mix garlic with salt and coat over salmon.

3.Place the salmon on herbs.

4.Place the pan in the grill and cook for 25 minutes.

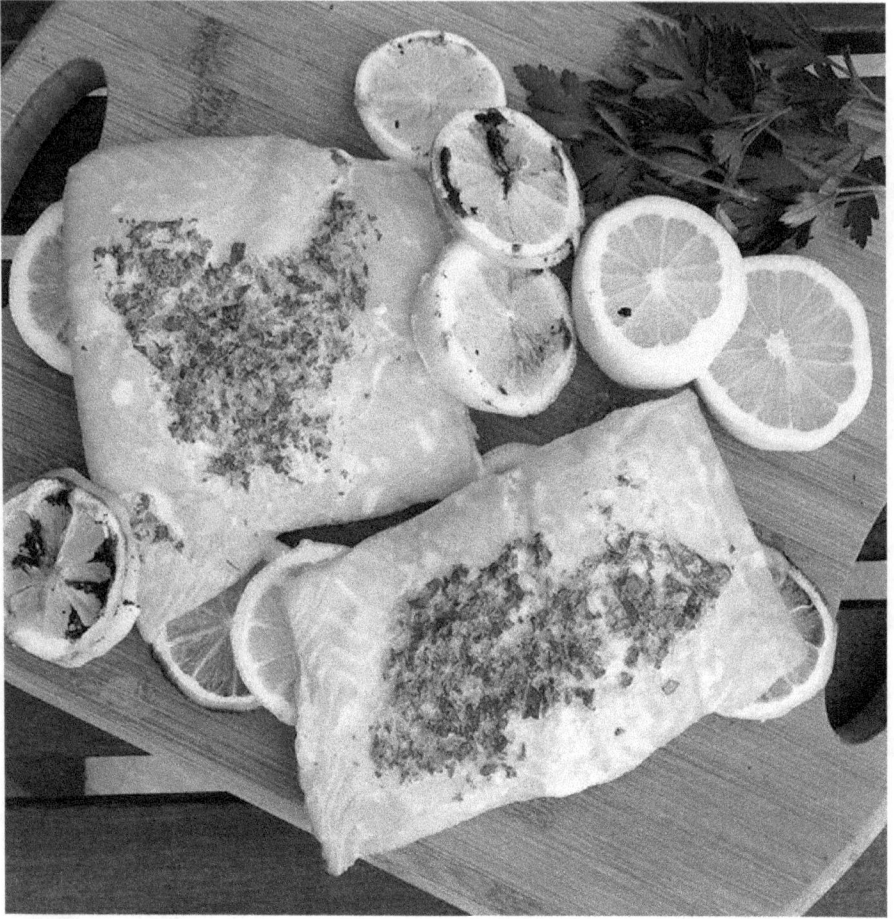

Herb-Baked Fish Fillets

Preparation time: 15 minutes
Cooking time: 15 minutes
Servings: 4

Ingredients:

Kosher salt to taste Black pepper to taste
2 tbsp butter
1/4 tsp dried thyme
1/4 cup corn flakes
1/4 cup of Onion
1/2 tsp dried tarragon
1 tsp chopped parsley
1 tbsp melted butter
1 lb fish fillets
One clove garlic (minced)

Directions:

1.Sauté garlic, onions, thyme, and tarragon in heated butter for two minutes.

2.Transfer the mixture over fish fillets.

3.Lightly sauté corn in butter and sprinkle salt and pepper to make cornflake crumbs.

4.Bake the fillets in an oven at 450 degrees for 15 minutes.

5. Serve and enjoy it.

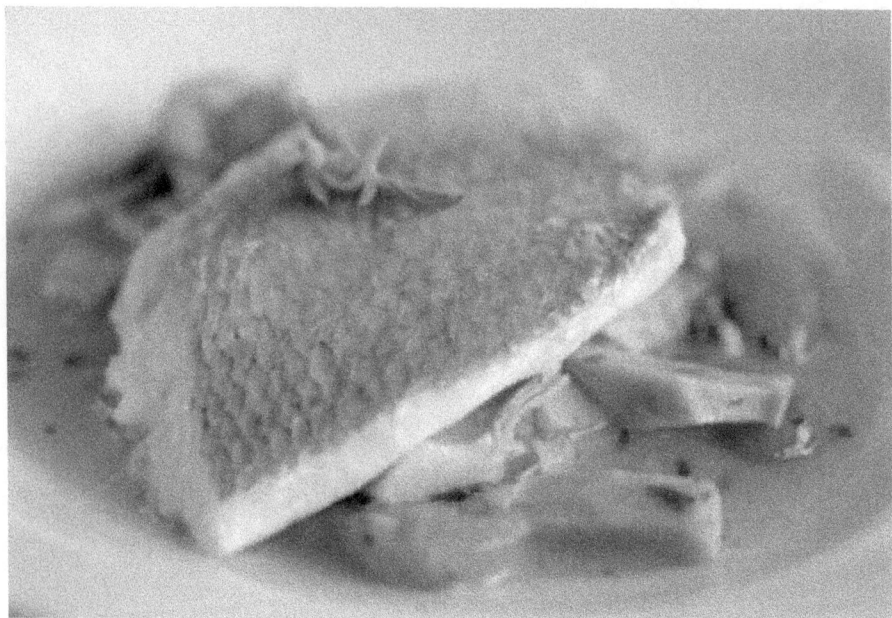

Japanese Salmon & Soba Noodle Salad

Preparation time: 10 minutes
Cooking time: 10 minutes
Servings: 4

Ingredients:

1/2 tbsp rice vinegar
1 tsp soy sauce
2 tbsp canola oil and 2 tsp sesame oil
200 g snow peas sliced
250 g soba noodles
Three salmon fillets
Four green onions sliced
60 g baby spinach leaves

Directions:

1.Bake the fillets wrapped in foil in a preheated oven at 180 degrees for five minutes.

2.Cook peas in boiling water for about 2 minutes and drain them.

3.Now cook noodles in the same water for five minutes.

4.Now mix everything in a bowl and serve.

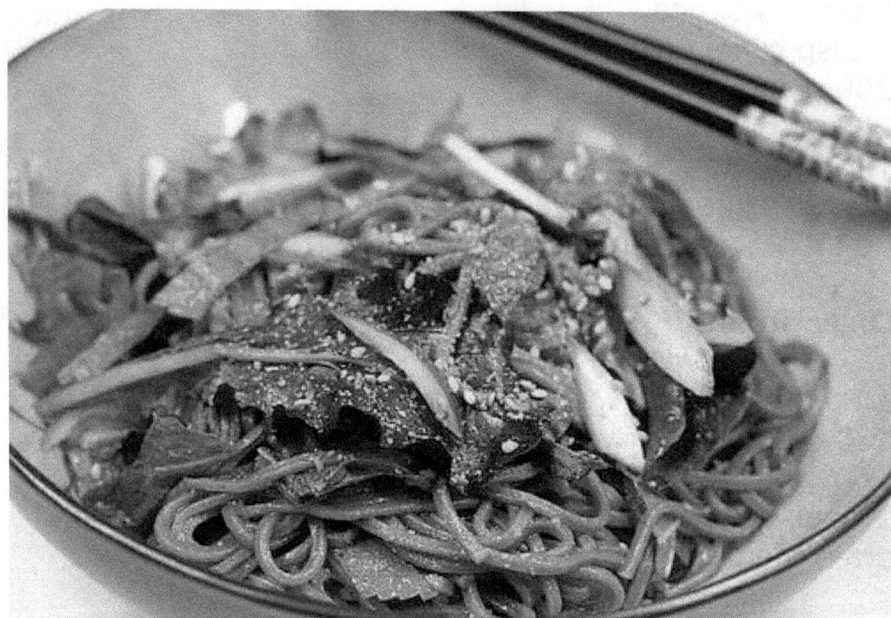

Walnut-rosemary crusted salmon

Preparation Time: 15minutes
Cooking Time: 0 minutes
Servings: 4

Ingredients:

Teaspoons Dijon mustard
¼ teaspoon lemon zest
1 teaspoon chopped fresh rosemary
¼ teaspoon of crushed red pepper
1 clove garlic, minced
1 teaspoon lemon juice
½ teaspoon honey
½ teaspoon kosher salt
1 teaspoon extra-virgin olive oil tablespoons panko
breadcrumbs tablespoons finely chopped walnuts
(1 pound) skinless salmon fillet, fresh or frozen
Olive oil cooking spray
Chopped fresh parsley and lemon wedges for garnish

Directions:

1.Firstly, preheat oven to 425 degrees F. Line a large
rimmed baking sheet with parchment paper.

2 Mix mustard, garlic, lemon zest, lemon juice,
rosemary, honey, salt and crushed red pepper in a
small bowl. Add panko, walnuts and oil in another small
bowl.

3 Put the salmon on the prepared baking sheet. Put the
mustard mixture over the fish and sprinkle with the
panko mixture, pressing to adhere. Lightly coat with
cooking spray.

4 Start baking until the fish flakes easily with a fork, about 8 to 12 minutes, depending on thickness.

5 Scatter parsley and serve with lemon wedges, if desidered

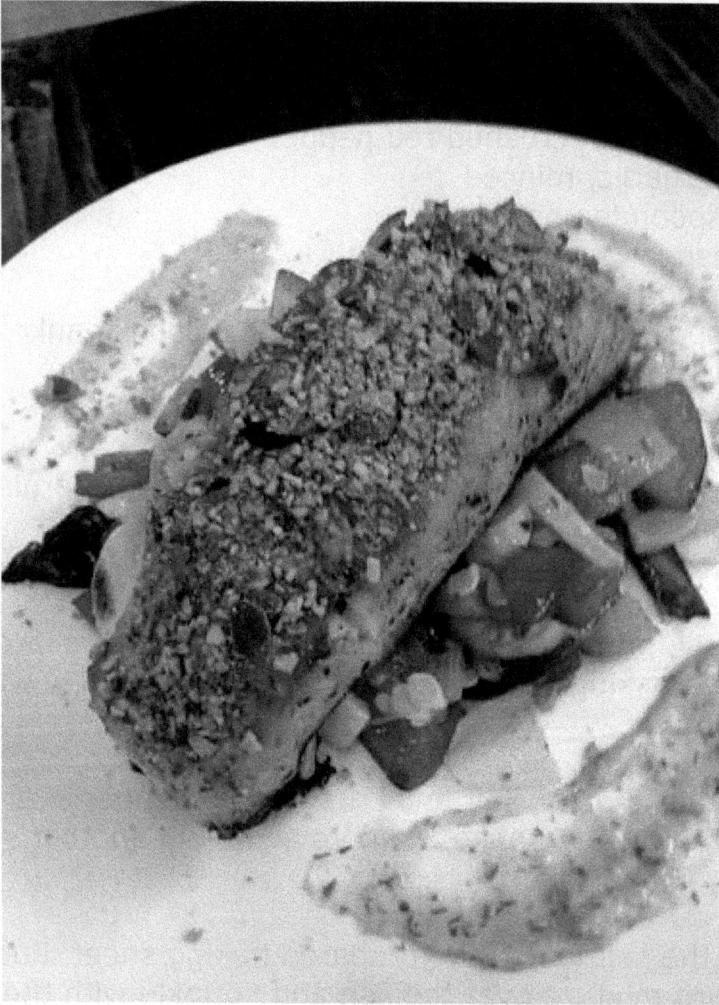

Turmeric chicken noodle soup recipe with noodles

Preparation Time: 1 hour
Cooking Time: 30 minutes
Servings: 2

Ingredients:

1 lb. chicken breast
cups chopped celery (stem only)
cups diced carrots
Salt and pepper
1 large onion, diced
large zucchinis, julienned into thin noodles
1 T ground turmeric
Fresh parsley, to garnish

Directions:

1.Put chicken breast, diced onions, chopped celery, and diced carrots in a large pot. Cover with water and bring to a boil, then cook until chicken breast is cooked through (about 30 minutes). Chicken is cooked when the juices run clear when you slice into it.

2. Now, transfer the chicken to a plate and let it cool before shredding it into pieces. Add ground turmeric to the soup, then turn heat down to medium-low. Let it simmer for 20 minutes until vegetables are soft.

3.Put in zucchini noodles and cook for 5 minutes. Divide zucchini noodles and soup into two bowls. Top with shredded chicken and garnish using fresh parsley.

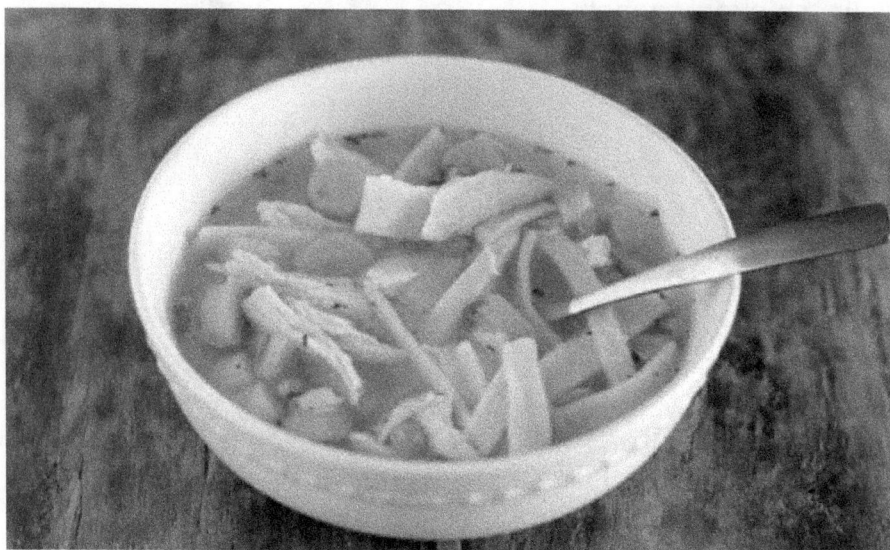

Paleo vegan BBQ meatballs

Preparation Time: 55 minutes
Cooking Time: 0 minutes
Servings: 24

Ingredients:

Tablespoon grapeseed oil
1 eggplant, skin on, diced 1 zucchini, diced
1 bell pepper, any color
½ cup walnuts, diced very fine and 1/2 cup paleo BBQ
sauce

Directions:

1.Take a baking sheet out with parchment paper and preheat oven to 350 degrees. In a large pan, heat grapeseed oil. Add pepper, eggplant, walnuts and zucchini.

2.Sautee until browned, for about 15 minutes. Stirring regularly to prevent burning. Remove from heat and let cool for about 5 minutes.

3.Now, add to vitamin blender with tamper and grind until soft- making sure to use tamper to stir mixture. Remove your mixture from blender and put into a larger bowl.

4.After that, take 1/4 cup mixture and roll into a tightly packed ball. Place on parchment paper lined baking sheet. Continue rolling balls. Bake at 350 degrees for 20 minutes, until they're deep brown. This step helps the meatballs "set", so don't skip it!

5.At this time, you can remove your meatballs and freeze them for another use. If eating immediately, place meatballs in a pan with a drizzle of grapeseed oil over medium heat. Brown on all sides, for about 8 minutes.

6.Mix BBQ sauce, stir well. Let sauce heat up- about 2 minutes. Remove from heat and serve immediate

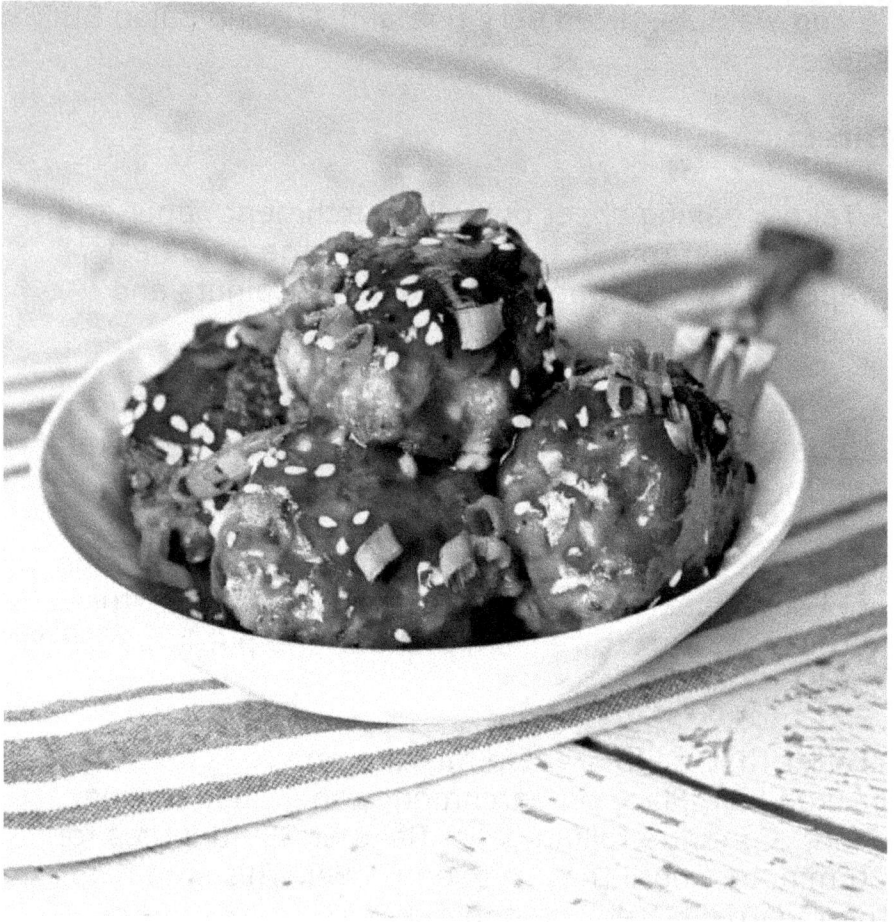

Turmeric sautéed greens

Preparation Time: 3 min
Cooking Time: 0 minutes
Servings: 3-4

Ingredients:

1 tablespoon olive oil
1 2-inch piece fresh turmeric
1/4 teaspoon kosher salt garlic cloves, minced
tablespoons water
Bunches kale, spinach, or Swiss chard, thinly sliced

Directions:

1 Firstly, heat oil in a large sauce pan by using medium heat.

2 Now, add garlic and turmeric and sauté for 30 seconds.

3 Further, add kale and salt and sauté for 1 minute.

4 Finally, add water to the pan and cook stirring until the greens are just wilted and serve.

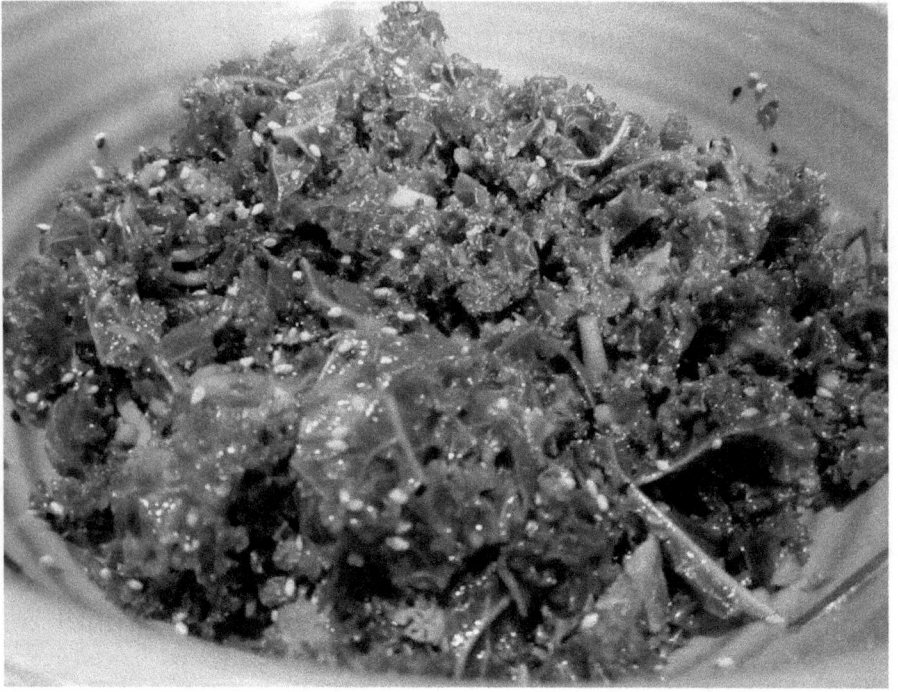

Cauliflower rice

Preparation Time: 15 minutes
Cooking Time: 5 minutes
Servings: 1

Ingredients:

Tablespoons olive oil
1 yellow or orange bell pepper
1 head cauliflower
1 onion, finely diced
2 cups fresh spinach, roughly chopped and 1 cup shelled edamame
1/2 teaspoon kosher salt teaspoons fresh ginger, minced tablespoons low sodium soy sauce scallions, chopped

Directions:

1.Firstly, heat a large wok or sauté pan over medium heat, add oil and sauté onion and ginger for 1 minute. Put bell pepper and cook for 1 minute.

2.Now, add the cauliflower and cook for an additional 2-3 minutes. Add spinach, edamame, soy sauce and salt. Cook for 4 minutes until the cauliflower is tender.

3.Finely, top with chopped scallions and serve.

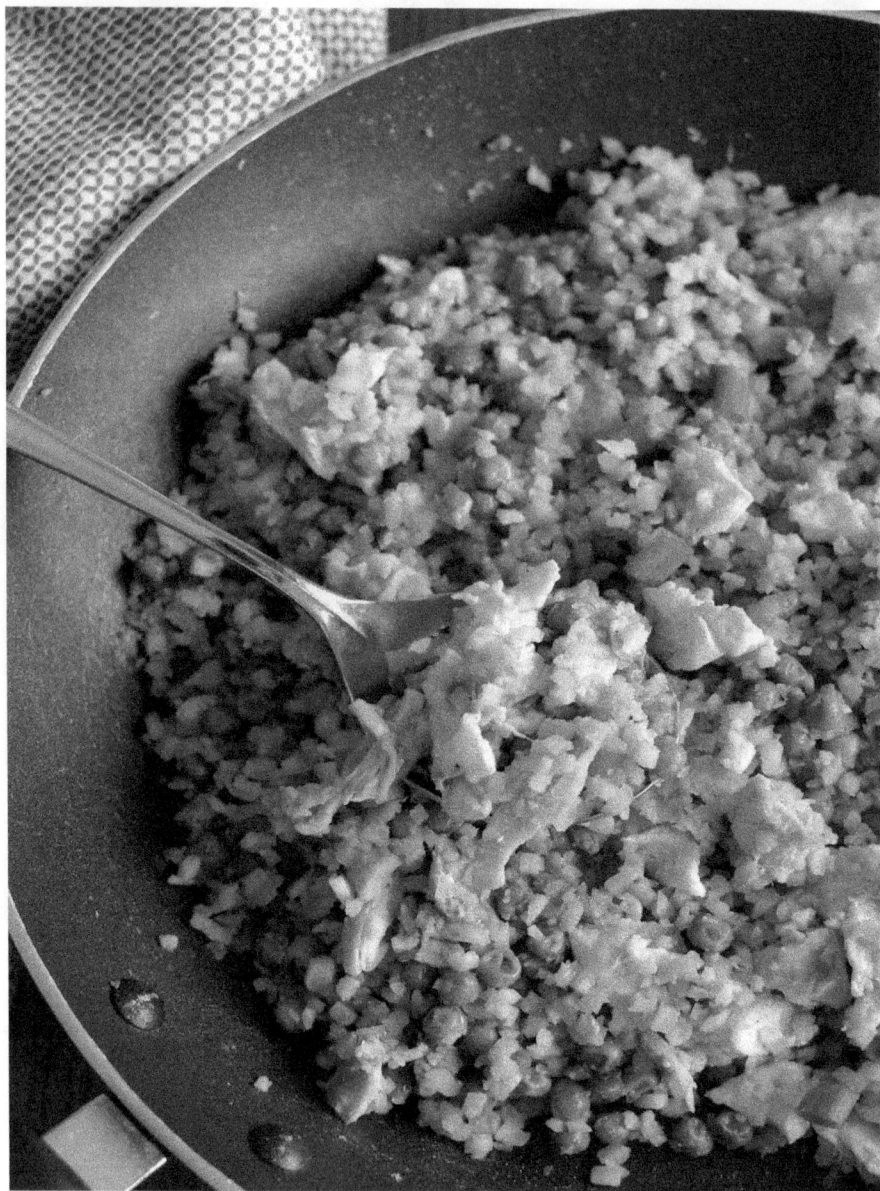

Seafood stew

Preparation Time: 40mins
Cooking Time: 30 minutes
Servings: 4-6

Ingredients:

1 tablespoon oil garlic cloves, minced
1 teaspoon kosher salt
1 cup dry white wine
1 large onion, diced
1 bay leaf
1 28-ounce can dice tomatoes
1/2-pound clams
1/2-pound shrimp, peeled and deveined 1/2-pound
shrimp, peeled and deveined 1 cup clam juice
1/2-pound mussels
1/4 cup minced parsley (optional)

Directions:

1.Take a large pot, heat oil by using medium heat.

2 Put the onions and cook for 3-4 minutes, until tender.
Add garlic and sauté for another minute.

3 Now, add the wine, tomatoes, clam juice, bay leaf and
salt. Bring to a boil, then reduce heat and simmer for
20 minutes.

4 Further, put in all the seafood at once and stir. Cook
until the shrimp is pink and mussels and clams have
opened, about 5-7 minutes.

5 Finely, Garnish with parsley if desired and serve immediately

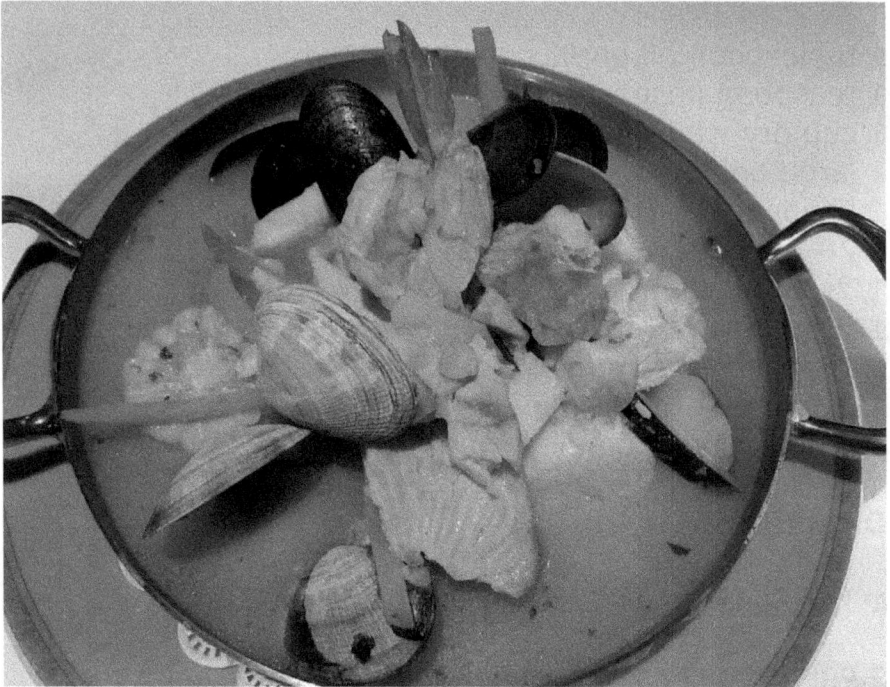

www.ingramcontent.com/pod-product-compliance
Lightning Source LLC
Chambersburg PA
CBHW050749030426
42336CB00012B/1727